The Complete Guide to Brain Health Supplements

By Lee Euler

And the Editorial Staff of *Brain Health Breakthroughs*

The Complete Guide to Brain Health Supplements
By Lee Euler
With Contributing Editors Carl Lowe, Michael Sellar, and Amanda Foxcroft

Published by Online Publishing & Marketing, LLC

IMPORTANT CAUTION:

The author of this Special Report is not a physician, doctor or professional health caregiver and this book is not intended as personal medical advice. It is a work of journalism and is intended to share the author's findings as a researcher and reporter. By reading this report, you are demonstrating an interest in maintaining good and vigorous health. This report suggests ways you can do that but – as with anything in medicine – there are no guarantees. You must check with private, professional medical advisors to assess whether the suggestions in this report are appropriate for you – or you must accept full responsibility if you decide not to do so. Nothing in this report is meant to constitute personal medical advice for any particular individual.

The authors, editors and publishers of this report are not responsible for any adverse effects or results from the use of any of the suggestions, preparations or procedures the report describes. As with any medical treatment, the results described in this report will vary from one person to another. The authors, editors and publishers believe the information in this report is accurate but they cannot guarantee its accuracy.

ISBN 978-1-5323-6844-8

©Copyright 2018 by Online Publishing & Marketing, LLC, P.O. Box 1076, Lexington, VA 24450

All rights reserved. No part of this publication may be reproduced, stored in a retrieval system, or transmitted in any form or by any means, electronic, mechanical, photocopying, recording or otherwise, without the prior written permission of the copyright owner.

Printed in the United States of America

ABOUT THE AUTHOR

Lee Euler has written about natural health options for more than 20 years. His books and articles have been read by millions. He is the producer of the acclaimed video series *Awakening from Alzheimer's: The Event*. In addition, he's the Executive Director of the prestigious Alternative Cancer Research Institute, editor and publisher of three newsletters, *Brain Health Breakthroughs*, *Cancer Defeated*, and *Aging Defeated*, and the author of numerous books and reports including *The Missing Ingredient for Good Health*, *Don't Touch My Prostate*, *The Oxygen Miracle*, and *Breast Cancer Cover-Up*. He has contributed to publications of many top doctors including Julian Whitaker, David Williams and William Campbell Douglass, Health Sciences Institute, and others.

Contents

Acetyl l-Carnitine... 1

Anthocyanins 3

Ashwagandha 6

B Vitamins.. 8

B12 11

Bacopa 15

Beetroot... 16

Berberine 18

Vitamin C 20

Caffeine... 22

Carnosine 24

Chocolate 26

Choline 32

Cinnamon 38

Coconut Oil, MCT Oil 41

Curcumin and Turmeric 44

Vitamin D 46

Vitamin E 52

Ecklonia cava 56

Fisetin 58

Fish Oil 61

Gallic Acid 63

Garlic 65

Gastrodin 67

Ginkgo biloba 69

Glutathione... 71

Gotu kola.. 74

Grape Seed Extract 76

Green Tea 77
Huperzine A 85
Vitamin K 87
Lemon Balm 89
Lion's Mane Mushroom 91
Lithium 96
Luteolin 99
Magnesium 101
Melatonin 103
Mushrooms 105
NAC (N-Acetyl-L-Cysteine) 108
Phosphatidylserine (PS) 110
Pomegranate 112
Probiotics 114
Pterostilbene 117
Rhodiola 120
Rosemary 122
Saffron 124
Sage 126
SAMe 128
Selenium 130
Skullcap/Baicalin 134
Spermidine 136
Sulforaphane 137
Theanine 140
Vinpocetine 141
Xanthohumol 144
Zinc 146

Acetyl l-Carnitine

Imagine your brain is like a hot new nightclub... everyone wants to get in, but only a select few – like celebrities – are actually allowed in.

Your "blood-brain barrier" – as doctors call it – is just like the red velvet cord that allows the VIPs into a club and keeps everyone else out. The blood-brain barrier allows only water and a selective crowd of nutrients to pass. Its purpose is to keep out substances that might harm the brain, but sometimes it keeps out helpful nutrients and medications as well.

Now studies show that one "celebrity" nutrient – **acetyl-l-carnitine** – has exclusive access to the brain and can reverse dementia, improve memory, and even treat Alzheimer's disease. Another form of this nutrient, l-carnitine, can't get past the velvet rope. So if you don't take the right form, it can be the difference between health and dementia.

Confirming this celebrity status, dozens of studies all agree: acetyl-l-carnitine is one of the few molecules allowed through the highly selective blood-brain barrier because it is fat soluble. And that ability might make it particularly useful for treating Alzheimer's disease.

Acetyl-l-carnitine (or ALC) is primarily an energy booster. It helps transport fatty acids into a cell's mitochondria, the cell's "batteries" or "power plants" which can burn oils for energy. ALC is also known to help repair damaged mitochondria, while reversing both mental and physical fatigue.

When ALC gets into the brain, it turns into a disease-fighting superhero.

Exciting news for Alzheimer's patients

Even though scientists have been intensively studying Alzheimer's disease for nearly 40 years, they're still not sure what causes the affliction.

One of the many theories is that inflammation and excess toxic build-up cause the development of the amyloid plaques and tau tangles that interfere with brain processes. If true, then ALC's ability to enter the brain as a powerful antioxidant is good news indeed.

One animal study showed that ALC, in comparison with its cousin l-carnitine, decreased dangerous oxidation in the brain – including reducing free radicals that are a byproduct of fat metabolism, and fighting inflammation.[1]

It's important to note that while some sources might use "l-carnitine" and "acetyl-l-carnitine" interchangeably, they're not the exact same molecule. ALC can penetrate the blood-brain barrier; l-carnitine cannot. You need to make sure you take acetyl-l-carnitine.

---

1 http://www.ncbi.nlm.nih.gov/pubmed/15591009

Another animal study revealed ALC increases synaptic neurotransmission (or how quickly your brain can process information) and improved learning capacity.[2]

And an experiment with 334 human Alzheimer's patients showed those under 61 years old gained significant benefits. Their ALC supplements actually slowed the progress of the disease![3]

Finally... and most importantly... ALC was shown to practically wipe out tau tangles and suppress development of the precursors to amyloid plaques.[4]

If this incredible discovery can be confirmed, this supplement could come to be regarded as a major treatment for Alzheimer's.

These studies are very exciting for Alzheimer's patients!

How to supplement with acetyl-l-carnitine

Most healthy people aren't necessarily deficient in ALC, because the body synthesizes it in the liver and kidneys. However, taking a daily 500 to 1500 mg supplement with food could be beneficial for preventing Alzheimer's disease.

Short-term studies on patients with Alzheimer's have been known to use up to three grams (3000 mg) per day, taken throughout the day. Check with your physician before taking such a large dose. It's not recommended that pregnant and breastfeeding women take ALC because the effects haven't been studied.

Remember, acetyl-l-carnitine is primarily responsible for increasing mental and physical energy. If you decide to supplement with ALC, be prepared for a boost!

You would have known about this valuable brain supplement as much as six years ago if you'd read our Special Report *Awakening from Alzheimer's*. In this one-of-a-kind collection of cutting edge Alzheimer's discoveries, author Peggy Sarlin covers the top foods and supplements for preventing or curing dementia and memory loss.

Peggy wrote *Awakening from Alzheimer's* with the advice of nine maverick doctors who are successfully reversing this disease that conventional medicine thinks is incurable.

---

2 http://www.ncbi.nlm.nih.gov/pubmed/20590847
3 http://www.ncbi.nlm.nih.gov/pubmed/9677506
4 http://www.ncbi.nlm.nih.gov/pubmed/21978079

Anthocyanins

Anthocyanins are a family of red, orange, blue and purple pigments – produced by plants to help them resist environmental hazards – that possesses enormous benefits for human health. These colorful plant nutrients have been documented to protect against cancer, heart disease, diabetes, infectious diseases, and more.

And over the last decade it's become clear that such colorful plant chemicals are also neuro-protective, offering resistance against Alzheimer's and Parkinson's disease.

Here's just a taste of what **anthocyanins** can do for you. (Oh, and anthocyanins and flavonols are two classes of natural plant chemicals collectively known as flavonoids. But don't worry too much about the terminology, it's technical and confusing.)

A large study involving 130,000 men and women over a 22-year period found that men who consumed the most flavonoids enjoyed a 40% reduced risk of developing Parkinson's disease compared to those who consumed the least.[5]

There was no such relationship for women. However, when the anthocyanin category of flavonoids was examined, both men and women had a lower risk of developing the brain disease.

Lead scientist Xiang Gao, M.D., Ph.D., said "…our findings suggest that a sub-class of flavonoids called anthocyanins may have neuroprotective effects."

The brain-protecting power of blueberries

Anthocyanins give a deep rich color to many fruits and vegetables, but are particularly abundant in berries. The most researched of these so far are blueberries.

Many laboratory and animal studies demonstrate that blueberries have cognitive benefits, protect against memory decline and can reduce amyloid-beta brain plaques. The first human trial in older adults who were at a greater risk of dementia confirmed that blueberries improve memory.[6]

The researchers said the anthocyanins in blueberries "have antioxidant and anti-inflammatory effects. In addition, anthocyanins have been associated with increased neuronal signaling in the brain centers mediating memory functions as well as improved glucose disposal, benefits that would be expected to mitigate neurodegeneration."

It's been shown that after a person drinks blueberry juice, the anthocyanins are found in the hippocampus and neocortex, which are regions of the brain essential for cognitive function.

---

5 https://www.ncbi.nlm.nih.gov/pubmed/22491871
6 https://www.ncbi.nlm.nih.gov/pubmed/20047325

In a rodent study, the anthocyanins in blueberries not only enhanced spatial memory but increased brain-derived neurotrophic factor (BDNF) in the hippocampus.[7] BDNF has been described as the fountain of youth for the brain, creating new neurons, promoting new connections and maintaining healthy cognitive function.

Many anthocyanin-rich foods to choose from

It's not all about blueberries. A number of other foods are now under investigation for their brain health properties.

Açai: These berries are known to have strong antioxidant properties thanks to high levels of anthocyanins. Rodent studies show that açai protects all areas of the brain from free radical damage and helps with 'neuronal housekeeping' by digesting and recycling damaged proteins.[8, 9]

Black Soybean: Cyanidin-3-glucoside is the most powerful of nine anthocyanins found in the seed coat of Cheongja 3, a selectively bred strain of black soybean. Researchers found them to have brain neuroprotective effects against free radicals. They described their study as significant because "this is the first report indicating potent health benefits of black soybean seed coat anthocyanins in neuroprotection."[10, 11]

Strawberry: A diet high in strawberries protected rodents[12] from age-related deficits in memory and learning, and a human study that looked at the diets of 16,000 participants over the age of 70 during a 20-year period concluded that "greater intakes of anthocyanins and total flavonoids were associated with slower rates of cognitive decline." The researchers found the most benefit came from eating strawberries and blueberries.[13]

Blackcurrant: This fruit is especially rich in anthocyanins. Dr. Derek Stewart from Scotland compared 20 fruits and found blackcurrants came out top in terms of antioxidant power. New Zealand researchers discovered in the laboratory that the anthocyanins in blackcurrants protect against Alzheimer's. Co-researcher Dr. James Joseph said, "I am confident the Alzheimer's protective effect we've seen will bear out in live humans."[14]

Aronia berries (chokeberries) contain abundant antioxidants and anthocyanins.

You won't find aronia berries in a grocery store (they also don't taste very good). That's why our sister company, Green Valley Natural Solutions, created an aronia berry extract called TheraFlex. It contains a very high level of anthocyanins in a convenient capsule.

---

7   https://www.ncbi.nlm.nih.gov/pubmed/23723987
8   https://www.ncbi.nlm.nih.gov/pubmed/19857073
9   http://www.nutraingredients-usa.com/Research/Acai-extracts-show-brain-health-potential
10 https://www.ncbi.nlm.nih.gov/pubmed/22491871
11 https://www.ncbi.nlm.nih.gov/pubmed/22575822
12 https://www.ncbi.nlm.nih.gov/pubmed/16837106
13 https://www.ncbi.nlm.nih.gov/pubmed/22535616
14 http://www.dailymail.co.uk/health/article-462802/Blackcurrants-berry-best-fruit-you.html

Tart cherry effects

Tart cherries are another fruit that is filled with intriguing anthocyanins.

The anthocyanins in tart cherry have been shown to relieve the pain of gout and arthritis, lower the risk of heart disease, help in the prevention and control of type 2 diabetes, bestow a better night's sleep and reduce muscle soreness after exercise. They may even reduce the risk of colon cancer.

And research shows tart cherries improve memory and cognition in adults who suffer from mild or moderate dementia.

Researchers have singled out tart cherries for their high concentrations of anthocyanins 1 and 2. These particular types can block COX-1 and COX-2 inflammatory compounds. Some pain medications like aspirin and ibuprofen work in much the same way.[15] In clinical tests, tart cherry performed about as well as these pain-killing OTC drugs, without the dangerous side effects such as gastrointestinal upset.

Because inflammation plays such a huge role in dementia, the anthocyanins in tart cherries amount to a nutritional treasure chest.

Michigan produces three-quarters of the tart cherry crop in the United States, so it's not surprising that neuroscientists led by Gary Dunbar at Central Michigan University decided to test tart cherry extracts on a mouse model of Alzheimer's disease.

They found that the mice taking the extracts (in combination with fish and emu oils) performed better on memory tests than those that didn't take the supplement. Brain autopsy showed a protective effect against inflammation and loss of neurons.

Prof. Dunbar said, "The major thing that we found out is that it has a real effect."

In the most recent study from Australia, conducted over a 12-week period, 49 men and women over 70, with mild-to-moderate dementia, drank either 200 ml (6¾ fluid ounces) a day of an anthocyanin-rich cherry juice or a control juice that had only a negligible amount of anthocyanins.

Only in the cherry group did the researchers find improvements in verbal fluency and both short and long-term memory. As a bonus, there was a significant reduction in blood pressure.

Tart cherries – the most common variety grown in the US is called Montmorency – can be consumed all year round because they are available dried, frozen, in juice or in concentrate.

If the foods mentioned are not on your shopping list, don't worry. Other anthocyanin-rich foods include asparagus, eggplant, red cabbage, purple cauliflower, purple onions, cranberries, elderberries, raspberries, plums, pomegranates, red fleshed peaches and grapes.

---

15 https://www.ncbi.nlm.nih.gov/pubmed/11695879

Although much is still unknown about how anthocyanins produce their protective effects, there is no doubting their health benefits.

Anthocyanin supplements are available, but in most cases many experts seem to believe that eating the anthocyanin-rich food or drinking the juice of these fruits and vegetables might be more worthwhile.

Let's leave the final word with Dr. Jeffrey Blumberg, senior scientist and director of the antioxidants research laboratory at Tufts University:

"While…the evidence is inadequate to define a specific dietary requirement, it's clear that consuming anthocyanin-rich foods should be encouraged."

Ashwagandha

It used to be a cliché of western movies: an old-time medicine show would feature a pitchman working to convince an audience of gullible locals that his tonic could cure practically everything. Resuscitate your sex life. Reduce your stress. Ease anxiety. Fight nasty diseases like cancer. Soothe a cranky ulcer.

If you heard that kind of talk today, you'd probably brush off the speaker as a snake oil salesman pushing a worthless product. But even though it sounds improbable, there actually is an herb from India that can do all these things, according to that country's medical experts.

And so far, nobody in a research lab has been able to prove them wrong.

Matter of fact, studies on this herb, which has been used in traditional Indian medicine for more than 6,000 years, show it can give you impressive brain and other health benefits that scientists are only beginning to understand.

An herb from the Ayurvedic tradition

The herb, called **ashwagandha**, is a widely used botanical employed in Ayurvedic medicine, the ancient healing tradition of India. Also called Indian winter cherry and Indian ginseng, ashwagandha is considered a "Rasayana," a medicinal plant known for its ability to make your mind and body function more effectively while lifting your mood.

Although more study is needed to understand exactly how ashwagandha helps the brain stay healthy, the study results so far have been impressive. When researchers gave ashwagandha to animals that suffered the kind of damage seen in Alzheimer's patients, they found proof that the herb can restore brain function elements that are destroyed when the brain starts to break down.

In one Japanese study, scientists worked with animals that had amyloid peptide accumulation in their brains. The growth of amyloid peptide occurs when Alzheimer's disease begins to affect memory. It makes up the brain plaques that are the main physical sign of the illness.

Just as sludge can block plumbing, amyloid peptides can gum up the brain's neural networks. They can eventually destroy your ability to navigate daily life.[16]

When these animals were given extracts from ashwagandha, the researchers discovered that the chemicals were converted into a substance called sominone that stimulated the reconstruction of brain structures. According to the scientists, it "significantly improved memory deficits… and prevented loss of axons, dendrites, and synapses."

Ashwagandha may help treat a wide range of other brain problems. In reviewing studies of the herb, researchers at the International Institute of Herbal Medicine in India emphasized, "There are dozens of studies that show that Ashwagandha slows, stops, reverses or removes neuritic atrophy and synaptic loss. Therefore Ashwagandha can be used to treat Alzheimer's, Parkinson's, Huntington's and other neurodegenerative diseases at any stage of the disease, even before a person has been diagnosed and is still in the state of mild forgetfulness."[17]

Also helps relieve stress, soothe ulcers and quench free radicals

Aside from these effects on the brain, a growing number of studies have shown that the natural chemicals in ashwagandha can support many other aspects of health. The herb helps protect mitochondria, the tiny structures that are often called the cell's energy factories.[18]

The herb has also been shown to offset the effects of stress and soothe stomach ulcers. At least part of its power, according to Indian scientists who have studied the plant, is due to its "potent antioxidant properties that help protect against cellular damage caused by free radicals."[19]

So you don't need a pitch man at a medicine show to see the benefits of ashwagandha. Its potential protective properties are known to be far-reaching and profound.

---

16 http://www.ncbi.nlm.nih.gov/pubmed/16553605
17 http://www.ncbi.nlm.nih.gov/pmc/articles/PMC3252722/?report=classic
18 http://www.ncbi.nlm.nih.gov/pubmed/2963652/
19 http://www.ncbi.nlm.nih.gov/pmc/articles/PMC3252722/?report=classic

B Vitamins

First, the bad news: As you grow older, your brain inevitably shrinks. At the same time it shrinks, the brain loses chunks of its mental capacity. And – no big surprise here – the smaller your brain, researchers believe, the fewer neuronal networks you have to work with when you are trying to create memories or deal with tasks that require intelligence.

So, your brain is slowly decreasing in size as you age. Now for the good news:

Although it's a challenge to keep your brain from growing smaller, researchers have found that B vitamins can slow the size reduction and, in the process, reduce your risk for the type of severe memory loss that occurs during Alzheimer's disease.

Brain sizing

The medical journal *PLOS One* published a two-year study of more than 150 senior citizens over the age of 70. The researchers found that those taking a supplement containing 500 mcg of B12, 20 mg of B6 and 0.8 mg of folic acid experienced, on average, much less brain shrinkage than did those in a no-vitamin control group.

Impressively, the researchers found that the brain regions the vitamins protected included the areas where reduction in size is linked to Alzheimer's disease – namely, a section called the entorhinal cortex and another called the hippocampus. On average, the B vitamins limited shrinkage during a two-year period to just one-half of one percent, a rate that fits within the normal range of aging. The people in the study who didn't get the vitamins averaged a brain loss of 3.7 percent.[20]

All of the 150 seniors in this study had already been suffering mild cognitive impairment, a memory problem that signals greatly increased risk of developing full blown Alzheimer's.

"This is strongly indicative that the B vitamins may be substantially slowing down or even potentially arresting the disease process in those with early stage cognitive decline. This is the first treatment that has been shown to potentially arrest Alzheimer's related brain shrinkage," says researcher David Smith of Oxford.[21]

The following chapter has a detailed report on one of the three vitamins in this study, B12, because it's so important. Meanwhile, let's take a close look at a B3, a vitamin the *PLOS One* study overlooked…

---

20 http://www.plosone.org/article/info%3Adoi%2F10.1371%2Fjournal.pone.0012244
21 http://www.nutraingredients.com/Research/High-dose-B-vitamins-help-prevent-Alzheimer-s-says-researchers

B3 boasts big brain benefits

For a glimpse of the possible benefits of B3, consider this story:

"...it took just under four months for us to see what seemed to be a full cure, but we started to notice improvement even after a few days."

So reported K.H. of Las Vegas in December, 2013. Her mother, suffering from dementia, was unable to tell you her age or what year it was. Yet in just a few short months her mental faculties made a full comeback.

Her mother said the experience "was like having windows suddenly flung open, like she could suddenly see things again that had been hidden from her."

And yet all it took to restore her to full mental health was a B3 supplement - a nutrient available in various forms including nicotinamide, niacinamide, nicotinic acid or niacin.

Nicotinamide in the treatment of Alzheimer's can be traced back to 1943, when Dr. William Kaufman published important findings. He said that patients who were deficient in the nutrient exhibited mental symptoms. This isn't surprising when you consider that a severe shortage of B3 causes pellagra, a deficiency disease characterized by dementia.

Dr. Kaufman reported that a lesser deficiency, while not severe enough to bring on pellagra, did cause impaired memory, poor concentration, inability to complete tasks, anxiety and quarrelsome behaviors. When patients supplemented with nicotinamide, the symptoms "disappeared....or improved considerably."

Low dietary intake puts you at severe risk

More recently, 3,718 people in the Chicago area, aged 65 or older and dementia-free, took part in a nine-year study. The researchers analyzed their diets and took note of decreasing mental abilities if any developed.

After three years, clinical evaluations were performed on a randomly selected subgroup of 815. 131 of them were diagnosed with Alzheimer's (an alarming statistic in itself). The researchers found that those with the lowest intake of B3 – 12.6 mg a day – were 80% more likely to receive a diagnosis of Alzheimer's compared to participants with the highest intake of 22.4 mg a day.[22]

After six years the researchers looked at the larger group and found those with the highest intake had 44% less cognitive decline than did those whose intake was the least.

---

22 http://www.ncbi.nlm.nih.gov/pubmed/15258207

"...a safe treatment for Alzheimer's Disease..."

In a study which used mice genetically engineered to develop Alzheimer's, those that took high doses of nicotinamide in their drinking water over four months performed just as well in memory tests as normal mice. Normal mice supplemented with B3 also performed better than did a control group of non-engineered mice fed only their usual diet.[23]

The study concludes: "These preclinical findings suggest that oral nicotinamide may represent a safe treatment for Alzheimer's disease..."

Lead researcher Dr. Kim Green didn't leave the matter in doubt: "The vitamin completely prevented cognitive decline associated with the disease, bringing them back to the level they'd be at if they didn't have the pathology. Nicotinamide has a very robust effect on neurons."

His colleague Frank LaFerla added, "It actually improved behavior in non-demented animals too. This suggests that not only is it good for Alzheimer's disease, but if normal people take it, some aspects of their memory might improve."

Clear benefits on many levels

Nicotinamide was a successful treatment in the study because it reduced levels of tau protein, one of the proteins associated with Alzheimer's. It also strengthened microtubules, the highways in neurons where information travels, helping to keep the brain cells alive. The death of these cells leads to dementia. Nicotinamide makes these highways wider and more stable.

Nicotinamide belongs to a class of compounds called HDAC inhibitors. These have protective effects on the central nervous system.

The first human trial of nicotinamide shows that the substance is safe to take and increases compounds in cells that help mitochondria produce energy while defending against stress and damage to DNA.

The study is available at https://www.nature.com/articles/ncomms12948. There is really no need to wait for further results. The vitamin has been used for over 60 years with safety.

The usual dose is 1000 mg three times daily. Some people suffer nausea at this level and have to cut the dosage in half. In rare cases nausea may continue at the lower dose. The reaction means the liver cannot handle the niacin supplement and the supplement should only be given under medical supervision.

If you do choose to take B3, make sure you read the label carefully. It is important to take the amide form – nicotinamide or niacinamide and NOT nicotinic acid or niacin. Not only did the research above use the amide forms, but pure niacin/nicotinic acid often causes an unpleasant skin reaction called "flushing".

---
23 http://www.ncbi.nlm.nih.gov/pubmed/18987186

The best food sources are eggs, tuna, chicken, turkey, crimini mushrooms, salmon, beef liver and kidney, asparagus, tomatoes and bell peppers.

B12

"It was as though a blanket of fog was lifted from her brain, and her personality reappeared."

So commented the relative of an 83-year-old woman who overcame dementia. She can now live independently, enjoy an active social life, and reads books in three languages!

All her mental health issues were resolved by restoring tissue levels of vitamin B12. Deficiency of this nutrient is common. According to some estimates it could affect up to 40% of the population and even more among the elderly. So it's of paramount importance to make sure you get enough. B12 is critical for neurological function and blood formation – so much so that's it should be considered "medicine" for dementia patients.

Vitamin B12 helps to make red blood cells and is vitally important to the healthy functioning of the nervous system. An extreme deficiency causes pernicious anemia – what some people used to call "tired blood" back in the day.

This type of anemia can give rise to serious neurological – i.e. brain – problems. It develops when the cells that produce a type of protein in the stomach called intrinsic factor are destroyed. You need intrinsic factor to absorb B12.

But recent studies make it clear that even when the body still provides its own intrinsic factor, up to four out of ten of Americans could still be at risk from less-than-adequate levels of vitamin B12. And the older you are, the more likely you are to suffer from a deficiency.

One study found that people with less than ideal B12 levels don't perform as well on memory and cognition tests and are also more likely to have shrinkage of the brain, one of the physical features of dementia. For some people, the symptoms of B12 deficiency can be similar to Alzheimer's.

Another study concluded that because of "the high prevalence of biochemical evidence of low vitamin B12 status in the elderly, steps should be taken to identify this condition, and to discover and treat its cause to avoid rapid cognitive decline."[24]

So the message is clear: Don't accept a diagnosis of Alzheimer's disease before having your B12 status tested.

---

24 https://www.ncbi.nlm.nih.gov/pubmed/22788704

And that's not all you should be tested for...

Anemia increases risk of dementia by 60 percent!

A recent study suggests older adults with anemia have an increased risk of dementia. Conducted over 11 years, the study included 2,500 men and women in their 70s. The researchers found a 60% increased risk of dementia for those who were anemic at the start of the study.[25]

The researchers believe anemia was the cause of dementia in these patients because of the low level of oxygen delivered to the brain. Because anemia affects as many as 23% of seniors – almost one out of four – this is an important finding.

The most common cause of anemia is a lack of iron, but a number of other factors can also bring on this condition.

Lead researcher Professor Kristine Yaffe said that "given how common both anemia and dementia are in older adults, more attention to the connection between the two is important, and I do think screening older adults for anemia makes sense."

Dr. Sam Gandy, director of the Mount Sinai Center for Cognitive Health in New York City, commenting on the study, was concerned that with Alzheimer's being a hot medical topic today, doctors will "be tempted to jump straight to that diagnosis" before running other tests that might reveal the patient has treatable, reversible causes of dementia.

The fact is, most cases of dementia are *not* caused by Alzheimer's disease. They're caused by prescription drugs, treatable nutritional deficiencies such as B12, anemia, reversible inflammation, sleep disorders and other causes.

If you have memory concerns, don't take the risk your doctor will be one of those who instantly reach for the dementia drug prescription pad. Make sure he tests for and rules out other explanations first. Insist on being tested. Your cognitive future may depend upon it.

B12 is difficult to absorb

It's a mistake to believe that only vegetarians can be low in B12 merely because this vitamin is found almost exclusively in animal foods. This isn't the case. Meat eaters can be deficient even when exceeding the recommended daily B12 intake of 2.4 micrograms.

That's because the absorption of B12 is a complex process that requires the digestive system to be in a very healthy state. It needs an abundant supply of hydrochloric acid and digestive enzymes along with intrinsic factor – the protein produced by the parietal cells of the stomach.

Inflammatory processes, bacterial overgrowth, disorders and diseases of the gastrointestinal system, or previous gastric surgery can all reduce absorption of B12.

---

25 https://www.ncbi.nlm.nih.gov/pubmed/23902706

Some medications can also lower the body's ability to take up B12. In particular metformin – prescribed for diabetes – is a problem. Also implicated in poor B12 absorption are the acid reflux or GERD drugs called proton pump inhibitors and H2-receptor antagonists.

Unfortunately, the symptoms of B12 deficiency are varied and can be hard to recognize or absent altogether. The most common signs are fatigue, "pins and needles," numbness, lack of muscle co-ordination, abnormal gait, 'brain fog', depression, memory loss and dementia. But there are many others. Doctors may not suspect a B12 deficiency from symptoms alone.

There are also limitations and shortcomings in the diagnostic tests used to assess B12 status. This means a person may suffer neurological signs of deficiency, yet have blood markers indicating B12 is in the normal range. Deficiency may not show up in any of the tests used.

These blood tests for nutrient levels should be taken with a grain of salt anyway. They can be valuable, but too often the "normal" ranges are merely the average levels for people in your age group. So if the average person is low in a given nutrient, it's considered "normal." And believe me, there are MANY nutrients in which the typical person in America and elsewhere is deficient.

Meanwhile the evidence that B12 deficiency increases the risk of developing dementia has been growing. Among the common vitamins and minerals we all know about – the ones that are typically found in multis – B12 has been shown to be the one most likely to reverse the symptoms of memory loss or mild cognitive impairment (MCI).

A study of 107 healthy people aged 61 – 87 gave these folks a battery of tests over a five-year period. Those with the lowest B12 status were over *six times more likely* to have brain shrinkage, a condition that is associated with dementia.[26]

"Many factors that affect brain health are thought to be out of our control, but this study suggests that simply adjusting our diets to consume more vitamin B12 through eating meat, fish, fortified cereals or milk may be something we can easily adjust to prevent brain shrinkage and so perhaps save our memory," says researcher Anna Vogiatzoglou.

In another study, an extensive array of memory tests, cognition tests and MRI scans were given to 121 people aged 65 or older. Those with the lowest B12 scored worse on the tests, had smaller brain volumes and less white matter, which indicates a loss of motor function.

Concerning these results, lead researcher Christine Tangney commented, "Every single marker of low vitamin B12 was correlated with low brain volume. If, as an older person, you start experiencing problems with memory, it would be smart for you to talk to your physician about whether you're getting enough B12 in your diet and through supplements."

---

26 https://www.ncbi.nlm.nih.gov/pubmed/18779510

Unexplained plunge in B12

While experts understand the importance of getting plenty of vitamin B12, precisely how this nutrient is used and regulated inside the brain remains mostly a mystery.

Research at Nova Southeastern University, in Florida, shows that the B12 level in the brain decreases in all of us as we age – *even as B12 blood levels remain about the same.* Brain levels drop so much, say these scientists, that the average senior citizen between the ages of 60 and 80 has only about one-third the amount of B12 in brain tissue found in a normal, healthy younger adult.[27]

The reason for this isn't clear. The researchers believe that it may be some sort of defense mechanism by the brain to deal with oxidative stress, a way to ensure proper genetic function in neurons as we get older, or it may be related to some sort of shift in metabolic function.

Note well, your doctor can only measure B12 levels in your blood, and these may not indicate whether your brain has enough. And he probably doesn't know this.

While we don't know what's going on with the brain's utilization of B12, there are studies that show taking supplements can protect against brain shrinkage with the passing years. And accelerated brain shrinkage has been linked to memory problems and other thinking difficulties.

Over 50? Supplements recommended

Because of the possible lack of symptoms and the difficulty of diagnosis, some researchers recommend all people over 50 take B12 supplements. The pills don't require the complex digestive processes that are needed when B12 is bound to food. B12 is also available as a patch absorbed through the skin or as a sublingual (under-the-tongue) tablet or spray.

All methods are effective. B12 is available in three forms, cyanocobalamin, hydroxocobalamin or methylcobalamin.

Integrative doctors almost always recommend the methyl form, as this is more metabolically active than the others. It may also be the only form that is effective. I take sublingual methylcobalamin myself, 1000 mcg every day.

Your body converts cyanocobalamin to methylcobalamin. So, in effect, when you take methylcobalamin, you're taking "predigested" B12 and it's absorbed much faster. Cyanocobalimin does get absorbed, albeit at a slower rate, so you can kind of look at cyanocobalamin as a "timed release" form of B12. People suffering from mild cognitive impairment may benefit from (and enjoy) the quicker jolt you get from taking the methyl form.

The 83-year-old woman mentioned earlier overcame dementia using the methyl form. When this was switched to the hydroxo form, her dementia returned. Reverting back to methylcobalamin restored her mental health.

---

27 http://journals.plos.org/plosone/article?id=10.1371/journal.pone.0146797

If you choose to take a B12 supplement, methylcobalamin is the preferred option as far as my team's research has been able to determine.

At the very least, everyone in middle age or older should take B12 supplements. You don't have to megadose, but about 1,000 mcg can be good health insurance. [28]

Bacopa

Centuries ago, ancient physicians discovered a plant growing in the brackish bog waters of India that contained some amazing therapeutic compounds.

The plant was *Bacopa monnieri* (also known as water hyssop, herb of grace, or Indian pennywort).

Originally used as a memory-enhancer, bacopa was found to greatly improve retention and memorization skills – which turned out to be highly beneficial for ancient scholars who needed to memorize long, intricate sacred scriptures and hymns.[29]

Besides memory, bacopa also improved attention span and cognitive processing, and helped develop a deeper retention of information.

This herb was so good at improving memorization and brain function that ancient physicians began using it to treat tribe members who suffered from insomnia and dementia.

Today, scientists are discovering the benefits of bacopa run even deeper than the ancients thought.

A natural brain booster

Bacopa acts as a neurological stimulant because it contains three very potent brain enhancers:

- Hersaponin – a compound that protects the delicate connections in the brain.
- Apigenin – a compound that supports the growth of new connections in the brain.
- Cucurbitacin – a potential anti-cancer compound.

These therapeutic compounds activate the brain's anti-inflammatory and antioxidant defenses as well as support natural brain health.

All these brain boosters do more than just increase function, however…

---

28 http://qjmed.oxfordjournals.org/content/102/1/17.long
29 http://www.wholehealthinsider.com/newsletter/nutrient-spotlight-bacopa/

Current studies using bacopa therapies are showing a drastic improvement in Alzheimer's patients, specifically with recognition of time, places, and people.

It worked for *all* these patients!

For six months, a test group of 39 Alzheimer's patients took 300 mg of an extract of *Bacopa monnieri* (called Bacognize®) twice daily.[30] After the study was completed, each patient took an aptitude test, and the results were astounding...

Just *two doses* of this natural remedy taken on a daily basis improved understanding, memory, language skills, and reading and writing skills in all patients participating in the test.

Each Alzheimer's patient in the study also reported drastic improvements in mood and quality of life.

Now that's amazing!

Getting the right dose...

How much Bacopa is needed to successfully prevent (or reduce the symptoms of) Alzheimer's disease?

Scientists will need to conduct more research to know for sure, but from what they know now, it appears a daily dose of 300 mg can improve brain function and memory. This refers to Bacognize, which is an extract of bacopa, not the whole herb. As always, consult your doctor before taking any medication or herbal supplements.

And if you'd like, you can grow bacopa – which flowers beautifully – in a hanging basket that gets plenty of sun.

Beetroot

"...it seems crazy not to eat it on a regular basis."

That's the view of UK-registered dietitian and TV nutritionist Carrie Ruxton. She was extolling the nutritional properties and wide-ranging health benefits of **beetroot** – a vegetable packed with fiber, vitamins, minerals and phytonutrients.

Consumed on a regular basis, it reduces inflammation, slashes your risk of cancer, lowers your blood pressure and increases your endurance.

And now researchers have started to look at its potential to boost brain health. They like what they're seeing.

---

30 http://www.academia.edu/1196726/Effect_of_Bacopa_monnieri_on_Cognitive_functions_in_Alzheimers_disease_patients

Experts believe the chief benefit of beetroot is its high level of dietary nitrate.

Once in the body, nitrate is converted to nitric oxide in the endothelium - the lining or inner surface of the arteries. Nitric oxide plays a fundamental role in vascular function by dilating blood vessels – meaning it provides a wider tube for the blood to pass through. This helps maintain healthy blood and oxygen flow throughout the body.

In 2011, a team of researchers from Wake Forest University, North Carolina, were interested in whether beetroot could increase cerebral blood flow.[31]

To this end, they split 16 volunteers with an average age of 75 into two groups. The participants were fed either 16 ounces of beetroot juice as part of a high nitrate diet, or had to follow a low nitrate diet. The study was conducted over four days.

Increases blood flow to the brain

Using scans, the researchers showed for the first time that a high nitrate diet increases blood flow to four areas of the frontal lobes – regions where blood flow diminishes with age. Loss of function in these parts of the brain is linked with cognitive decline and dementia.

In another study four years later, researchers from the UK enrolled 40 healthy men and women aged 18 - 27. The participants drank either 16 ounces of beetroot juice or a low nitrate placebo drink.[32]

90 minutes later they were given cognitive tasks while their brains were scanned. Increased blood flow to the frontal cortex and improved cognitive performance were seen in the beetroot group.

In the most recent study, again conducted at Wake Forest, the researchers wanted to see if the somatomotor cortex could be boosted by beetroot juice. This part of the brain processes messages coming from muscles. An established benefit of exercise is the strengthening of this area.[33]

The scientists were also interested in secondary connections between the motor cortex and the insula, which is involved a wide variety of processes including motor control and cognition.

The study involved 26 participants with an average age of 55. All of them had been diagnosed with high blood pressure. They were assigned to six weeks of moderate exercise three times a week. No one in the group was taking more than two medications a week for their condition. An hour before each exercise session they drank either beetroot juice or a low-nitrate placebo. Their brains were scanned at the end of the trial period.

---

31 https://www.ncbi.nlm.nih.gov/pmc/articles/PMC3018552/
32 https://www.ncbi.nlm.nih.gov/pubmed/26037632
33 http://www.medicalnewstoday.com/articles/316997.php

Results showed that the beetroot group had developed greater connectivity between brain regions to "more closely resemble that of younger adults..."

These findings were described by the Wake Forest team as "exciting" – and regular exercise coupled with beetroot juice could be important in maintaining brain health and mobility as we age.

The top nitrate foods

By far the best sources of nitrates in the diet are greens, butter and oak leaf lettuce, spring and beet greens, Swiss chard, bok choy, basil, coriander and parsley; all contain high amounts.

But the star is rocket salad (arugula) with 480 mg of nitrates per 100 grams.

While beets themselves contain a good amount of nitrate (110 mg per 100 grams), you need to consume them in the form of beetroot juice to enjoy the big dose of 279 mg per 100 grams that the drink contains. By eliminating the fiber, the juice provides a more concentrated dose of the nutrients.

If you do choose to go down this path, it's best to check first with your doctor, as regular consumption of beetroot juice may not be indicated in certain medical conditions.

Berberine

It's always exciting when modern medicine and scientific studies catch on to something Eastern medicine has known for thousands of years.

And now research has focused on **berberine** – a natural yellow dye that's been used for thousands of years for everything from fighting the plague in 14th century China to fighting modern diseases like diabetes, insulin resistance (prediabetes), and heart disease.

What's more, new studies also show this particular dye has incredible neuroprotective benefits … has been labeled a "medicinal alkaloid" … and could be the future of Alzheimer's prevention.[34] Alkaloids are a class of nitrogen-rich compounds found in plants.

Berberine is one of them. It comes from the roots of several plants, including barberry, goldenseal, Oregon grape, and goldthread, among others.

Beyond being used as a bright yellow dye in India, it's also a powerful antibiotic and has been implicated in treating high cholesterol, high blood pressure, leaky gut syndrome, immune system deficiencies, joint and bone problems, and multiple types of cancers.

---

34 http://www.sciencedirect.com/science/article/pii/S1002007109002883?np=y

Recently, berberine's ability to protect the brain, fight inflammation and oxidative damage, and even resist the onset of Alzheimer's is making waves in the scientific community.

According to a 2009 study from the *Biological & Pharmaceutical Bulletin*, berberine inhibits enzymes that create the amyloid beta proteins that build up and eventually create the plaques found in Alzheimer's dementia. The researchers noted that the alkaloids would "clearly have beneficial uses in the development of therapeutic and preventative agents for Alzheimer's disease and oxidative stress-related disease."[35]

Another review paper, published in 2011, showed how berberine fronts a multi-pronged attack by inhibiting three classic chemical channels involved in Alzheimer's disease. The remedy thereby fights inflammation in the brain and reduces amyloid plaque build-up.

A study from *Progress in Natural Science* confirmed that the plant extract does this by reducing the enzymes that create the amyloid beta proteins and physically unfolding the proteins, making them less "sticky" and preventing plaque formation.[36]

The researchers noted that benefits occurred with higher concentrations of berberine. The half-life of berberine in the body is approximately three to four hours. So it's generally considered safe to take the supplement three times a day to get maximum benefits.

Remember, berberine is a multi-benefit supplement. While its neuroprotective benefits are still under study, the evidence shows it definitely fights inflammation and cellular free radical damage, increases adiponectin expression to aid in body fat loss, and acts as a powerful antibiotic against fungal infections, yeasts, parasites, and bacterial or viral infection.

There are few reported side effects – it apparently doesn't bother most people – but berberine is not recommended for newborns or for women who are pregnant or nursing, because the effects on babies are simply unknown.

Berberine is widely used as a natural antibiotic and antiviral, and for this reason I have some concerns about its possible long-term effects on friendly intestinal bacteria. I would take berberine with a probiotic supplement to counter this potential problem.

And until we know more, I'm inclined to think berberine is appropriate mainly for people who have dementia or are at clear risk. I'm doubtful that healthy people should make long-term use of an antibiotic, even a natural one.

---

[35] https://www.ncbi.nlm.nih.gov/pubmed/19652386
[36] http://www.sciencedirect.com/science/article/pii/S1002007109002883?np=y

Vitamin C

Vitamin C more or less started the whole current wave of alternative health more than 50 years ago when Linus Pauling, a Nobel Prize winner, first told the world this vitamin could treat the common cold – and cancer, too.

That was many moons ago. It's easy to forget about vitamin C when looking for a brain supplement. Everyone knows about it (or so people think), and surely all of us are taking enough already.

What could possibly be new about this well-known nutrient? Quite a lot, it turns out.

Evidence of vitamin C's importance to the brain can be seen in the fact that brain cells latch onto vitamin C like their lives depend on it – and they do! That's why the concentration of vitamin C in the brain's neurons is 200 times higher than the concentration of vitamin C in your blood.[37]

Researchers believe that if you're missing out on vitamin C, then oxidative stress – an excess of free radicals – makes you much more liable to fall victim to Alzheimer's disease and other neurodegenerative conditions. As the number of free radicals grows, oxidative stress can kill neurons or make them malfunction.

Aging brains more likely to lose their C

Getting vitamin C to the brain is no simple task. While most animals can make their own vitamin C, human bodies can't. We have to eat it in food – or take supplements – and then vitamin C has to be taken out of the digestive tract and sent into the brain and other organs.

Part of the process of getting this nutrient to brain cells involves molecular carriers that transport vitamin C into the cerebrospinal fluid that flows into the brain. Another route works with transporters that carry vitamin C in the blood and move it to the blood-brain barrier where it is escorted into brain tissue.

The blood-brain barrier is supposed to be a one-way street for vitamin C, meant to keep most vitamin C from leaving the brain once it gets in. But researchers believe that as we age, the barrier's ability to retain the vitamin in brain tissue starts to falter, allowing the vitamin to seep out and the brain's levels of vitamin C to drop.

That being said, there is other intriguing evidence for vitamin C helping to protect the brain:

A study at Oregon Health & Science University shows that vitamin C seems to be necessary for basic neuron function. This conclusion grows out of studies of the ways in which

---
[37] https://www.ncbi.nlm.nih.gov/pubmed/10782126/

nerve cells in the eye require vitamin C.[38]

"We found that cells in the retina need to be 'bathed' in relatively high doses of vitamin C, inside and out, to function properly," says researcher Henrique von Gersdorff. "Because the retina is part of the central nervous system, this suggests there's likely an important role for vitamin C throughout our brains, to a degree we had not realized before."

The Oregon scientists point out that both the eye and the brain contain special receptors, called GABA-type receptors, that help control the rapid communication that takes place between brain cells.

Since the eye's GABA receptors malfunction when they don't have enough vitamin C, the researchers think it likely that GABA receptors throughout the brain need vitamin C to fulfill their proper functions.

However, vitamin C's functions in the brain are still not completely understood. But scientists do know this: If you suffer a vitamin C deficiency, your brain retains the vitamin in the brain longer than anyplace else in your body.

"Perhaps the brain is the last place you want to lose vitamin C," von Gersdorff says.

He adds that these findings may offer a clue as to why scurvy, the vitamin C deficiency disease, progresses the way it does. A primary symptom of scurvy is depression. That may arise from the lack of vitamin C in the brain.

Don't wait till you've got dementia to up your C

While vitamin C is crucial for keeping the fats in neurons and brain cell membranes from being oxidized, using vitamin C to fight conditions like Alzheimer's disease is not a straightforward process. When researchers have given vitamin C to people who already have Alzheimer's disease, they haven't found any benefit.

But when they look at people who consume vitamin C as they age – before memory problems have started – they have uncovered evidence that it may be a preventive that lowers the risk for Alzheimer's.

For example, a six-year study in the Netherlands looked at the brain health of more than 5,000 people over the age of 55. The researchers found that folks who consumed vitamin C supplements (as well as vitamin E) ran a much lower risk of developing Alzheimer's disease during the research.

In this study, the protective benefit of vitamin C supplements was particularly clear in the people who were smokers.[39]

---

38 http://www.ncbi.nlm.nih.gov/pubmed/21642435
39 https://www.ncbi.nlm.nih.gov/pubmed/12076218/

The research into vitamin C's brain health benefits makes it clear – the sooner you start eating plenty of fruits and vegetables and taking vitamin C supplements, the better off your memory will be. A study at Vanderbilt University concludes, "There is overwhelming evidence that a lifetime of good nutrition, thus avoiding sub-clinical deficiency in vitamin C and other antioxidants, is necessary to restrict the accumulation of damage."[40]

So don't wait. Put vitamin C to work for your brain today.

Caffeine

Most of us gulp down caffeinated drinks to give ourselves an energy lift and deal with the workload of everyday life. But for the plants that generate caffeine in the first place, it serves as a pesticide that drives away insects and animals that would like to munch on their leaves and fruit.[41]

In our bodies, caffeine stimulates the central nervous system and makes us more alert.

But scientists are finding that, beyond its stimulating effects, **caffeine induces the brain to make more of an enzyme that fends off Alzheimer's and other forms of dementia**.

According to researchers at the University of Indiana at Bloomington, the enzyme, known as NMNAT2 (nicotinamide mononucleotide adenylyl transferase 2 – just in case you need to know) helps improve the health of the brain in two crucial ways. . .

- It guards neurons from the destructive effects of stress.
- It keeps a protein called tau from folding the wrong way and forming masses of harmful plaques among the brain's neurons.[42]

Proteins in the body often have a complex geometry and have to fold in just the right way to keep cells functioning properly. Wrinkled up, misfolded proteins, say the Indiana scientists, are involved in diseases that disable neurons.

The misfolded proteins have been linked to neurodegenerative disorders such as Parkinson's and Huntington's diseases, and amyotrophic lateral sclerosis (ALS or Lou Gehrig's disease) as well as Alzheimer's.

Caffeine helps to keep those proteins straightened out and in the right configuration.

---

40 https://www.ncbi.nlm.nih.gov/pmc/articles/PMC3727637/
41 https://www.ncbi.nlm.nih.gov/pubmed/16781610/
42 https://www.ncbi.nlm.nih.gov/pubmed/?term=NMNAT2+caffeine

Reducing stress in brain cells

In another study, researchers in Portugal and France have shown that caffeine can keep your memory humming along in good working order as you get older by hooking up with a particular brain cell receptor. Left on its own, this receptor increases stress in brain cells and can slow your mental abilities as you age.[43]

The lab tests show that caffeine cools off the activity of this receptor, known as adenosine A2A, and keeps it from disrupting memory circuits in the brain's hippocampus and cortex.

Drinking more caffeine equals less Alzheimer's

The brain benefits of caffeine have also been confirmed by researchers who have looked at the brain health of older people who drink caffeinated drinks.

At the University of Wisconsin-Milwaukee, researchers found that among older women, those who consumed more than 261 mg of caffeine a day had a 36 percent reduced chance of developing dementia during the ten years of the study.[44]

261 mg is about how much caffeine there is in two or three 8-oz cups of coffee. 261 mg would also be found in about six 8-oz cups of tea or about eight 12-ounce cans of cola. These are all estimates. It depends on how strong you make your brew.

But don't drink those colas! The sugar in soft drinks is devastating for your health. Get your caffeine from an unsweetened source. (There are other harmful ingredients in colas, but that's another subject.)

Oh, and one last thing to keep in mind – once you get past those 261 mg, you don't get much more benefit from adding more caffeine to your day. For instance, a ten-year study in the Netherlands found that seniors who drank more than three or four cups of coffee didn't experience more brain health from every extra cup.[45]

So don't feel compelled to go overboard on caffeine. Taking too much of it can lead to excess feelings of anxiety, increase your heart rate and interfere with your sleep. I'm sensitive to caffeine, and one cup of coffee a day is about all I care to deal with. I'm plenty energized. If two or three cups are required, I'll have to find another brain booster.

Caffeine also stays in many people's systems much longer than they think. If you sleep poorly I strongly recommend cutting way back, or even cutting out coffee and tea altogether for a couple of weeks, then drinking less when you resume (not easy to do, I know).

---

43 https://www.ncbi.nlm.nih.gov/pubmed/27510168
44 https://www.ncbi.nlm.nih.gov/pubmed/?term=ira+driscoll%2C+caffeine
45 https://www.ncbi.nlm.nih.gov/pubmed/16929246

While caffeine may be helpful to the brain, good sleep is absolutely *essential*. Besides contributing to memory loss, inadequate sleep also increases the risk of cancer.

Carnosine

Could an unusual Asian bird with black bones be a source of carnosine – a nutrient that can protect your brain as you age? Respected researchers believe it can. And, luckily, you don't have to go searching for this exotic creature to reap the nutritional benefits contained in its muscle tissue. Brain-boosting carnosine is available much closer to home.

But first, back to the bird. As traditional Chinese medicine (TCM) becomes more accepted around the world, researchers are discovering areas where this Asian medical system overlaps with Western medicine. And sometimes these congruent areas of therapy occur in the oddest places.

A thousand years ago, the carnosine-rich meat of the Chinese bird called the black-bone silky fowl began to earn renown as an anti-aging tonic.

Aside from the health reputation of its meat, the bird is odd because beneath its snowy, white feathers are black colored skin, black meat and black bones.

Its strange appearance hasn't slowed its popularity in China. Eating this bird is believed to relieve menstrual cramps and postpartum disorders, lower the risk of diabetes, prevent anemia, improve muscle strength, boost brain power and generally fight aging.

No one really understood why this meat seemed to be so good for health until an analysis of its muscle tissue established that it is dense with carnosine, a peptide (protein component) that is already available as a dietary supplement in the U.S. You can buy it over the counter. No need to kill those poor birds.

In your body, carnosine collects in the brain and muscles. It is so versatile in promoting the health of so many parts of the body (including the brain) that researchers have been hard at work merely trying to figure out how it penetrates so many important organs. They're still not sure.

Brain savior

When it comes to protecting the brain against Alzheimer's and dementia, researchers have identified several ways carnosine can help.

One of its most important roles is the promotion of healthy mitochondria, the small structures in every cell (including brain cells) that produce the energy necessary for physiological functions. When you suffer brain maladies like Alzheimer's disease and Parkinson's disease, the mitochondria frequently begin to malfunction.

According to researchers in Italy,[46] carnosine "completely rescues AD (Alzheimer's disease) and aging-related mitochondrial dysfunctions."

When the scientists tested the effects of supplemental carnosine on lab animals that were suffering the rodent equivalent of Alzheimer's, they found that not only did the animals shrug off Alzheimer's, but their mitochondria began functioning at a higher capacity than those of animals that had never even had Alzheimer's!

If that works with humans, too, I believe I want to try it!

As the scientists are quick to point out, "The functional role of carnosine is still not completely understood…" But they note that it is a chelating agent that can remove harmful metals from the brain, as well as an antioxidant and free-radical scavenger that can intervene in oxidative harm to brain cells. (Free radicals are caustic substances that are blamed for many chronic conditions in the body. Antioxidants can neutralize their destructive action.)

Cell defense

Further research has shown that carnosine, in combination with other antioxidant nutrients, can protect the brain against the debilitating effects of stroke.[47] When researchers at the Medical College of Georgia gave carnosine along with blueberry, green tea and vitamin D3 to laboratory animals that had suffered strokes, they found the animals grew back new brain neurons at an accelerated rate.

"The numbers of new neurons found in the damaged brains of the treated (animals) was significantly higher," says researcher Paula Bickford. Ms. Bickford has also performed research in the elderly indicating that carnosine can improve thinking abilities as you age.[48]

Aside from its usefulness in defending your brain, carnosine may be able to help you fend off the viruses that cause colds and flu. Researchers think that it's the carnosine in chicken soup that is at least partly responsible for making it such a popular tonic for those felled by respiratory infections.[49]

---

46 http://www.ncbi.nlm.nih.gov/pmc/articles/PMC3058055/
47 http://www.ncbi.nlm.nih.gov/pubmed/18260778
48 http://www.ncbi.nlm.nih.gov/pubmed/24134194
49 http://www.ncbi.nlm.nih.gov/pubmed/20841992

Chocolate

When you think about chocolate, the first thing that crosses your mind may be its rich, delicious taste and creamy texture. But if you're a medical researcher, visions of chocolate-boosted brainpower may also dance in your head.

As sales of chocolate expand every year (about 7 percent annually in the U.S.),[50] scientists have expanded their studies into the ways chocolate improves the health of brain cells.

One of the most recent advances in our knowledge of chocolate and its benefits focuses on plant compounds called polyphenols. Scientists at Johns Hopkins have been particularly interested in how polyphenols known as catechins (also contained in green tea) influence the survival and growth of neurons in the brain.[51]

Those neurons, which are the highways and byways on which your memories and thoughts travel, need a protein called brain-derived neurotrophic factor (BDNF) in order to grow and survive. In fact, researchers are coming to see BDNF as an extremely important factor in brain health. Famous author Dr. David Perlmutter calls it "growth hormone for the brain."

The Hopkins researchers launched their investigations because they were trying to find ways to restore the cognitive powers of people with HIV. Victims of HIV suffer reduced levels of BDNF, and that deficiency is at the root of many of the problems they have remembering things.

In their studies, the Hopkins scientists discovered that the catechins in chocolate help protect neurons by increasing the production of BDNF. Importantly, the scientists found that these natural chemicals travel across the blood-brain barrier – important because not all nutrients can breach that border. This means that after you digest chocolate and these chemicals enter your bloodstream, they can reach the brain and contribute to neuron growth and function.

Blood flow to the brain is another key element required for vigorous mental ability. When the blood supply to the brain is blocked, your cognitive abilities can also be dammed up.

Here, too, chocolate has been shown to open the gates to better brain health. Research at the University of Nottingham, in the UK, has demonstrated that phytochemicals in dark chocolate can increase cerebral blood flow for up to three hours after you eat chocolate. These scientists also believe the blood-flow-boosting effect of chocolate is potentially useful for treating dementia and strokes.

According to researcher Ian Macdonald, professor of metabolic physiology at the University of Nottingham, "The demonstration of an effect of consuming this particular beverage (cocoa) on cerebral blood flow raises the possibility that certain food ingredients may be beneficial in increasing brain blood flow and enhancing brain function, in situations where

---
50 http://www.candyindustry.com/articles/85215-report—19-5-billion-in-chocolate-sales-and-20–growth-in-organic
51 http://www.springer.com/about+springer/media/springer+select?SGWID=0-11001-6-1386344-0

individuals are cognitively impaired such as fatigue, sleep deprivation, or possibly aging."[52]

A brain honed to a sharp edge on chocolate

Along with showing that chocolate sets the physiological stage for better brain health, researchers have tested chocolate eaters to see whether their improved physiology is reflected in sharper mental performance. They haven't been disappointed: Their tests have shown measurable increases in mental power.

In a study at the UK's Northumbria University, researchers recruited 30 people aged 18 to 35 and brought them into the laboratory for chocolate drinks and computerized assessments.[53]

On each visit to the lab, the participants had to complete tasks that analyzed how anxious they felt and measured their ability to perform mentally demanding tests. The results clearly showed that eating or drinking chocolate boosted their test results and eased their emotional distress.

Chocolate wins the prize

If you'd like more evidence for chocolate's brain benefits, consider a survey by researchers at St. Luke's-Roosevelt Hospital and Columbia University. They found that the countries of the world with the highest chocolate consumption win the most Nobel prizes per capita.[54] And a survey of Norwegians in their seventies demonstrated that those who consistently ate chocolate did better on word tests than did chocolate abstainers.[55]

Quite a number of factors lead to winning a Nobel Prize, so I wouldn't jump to any conclusions based merely on this study. But it sure is interesting!

Potential Alzheimer's treatment

Because chocolate increases blood flow to the brain, enhances oxygen uptake and improves cognition, some scientists believe it has great potential in preventing Alzheimer's disease.

Just for the record, I eat some dark chocolate every day. It's become my afternoon replacement for caffeine, which keeps me awake at night if I drink too much.

So for me, dark chocolate has become a practical energy booster. But I'm happy to take the brain benefits on board while I'm at it. And what's the source of the benefits?

---

52 http://www.medsci.org/press/cocoa.html
53 http://www.northumbria.ac.uk/sd/academic/lifesciences/resinn/bpn/bpnrccasest/?view=Standard
54 http://www.ncbi.nlm.nih.gov/pmc/articles/PMC3544694/
55 http://www.ncbi.nlm.nih.gov/pubmed/19056649

Among chocolate's natural chemicals, flavanols – a sub-class of the polyphenols I mentioned earlier – are nutrients believed to help boost your brain. The cocoa bean (also called the cacao bean) has a unique blend of these beneficial plant compounds, and a number of studies have looked into their effects.

About nine out of ten patients see improvement

When 60 older people – average age of 73 – drank two cups of flavanol-rich cocoa each day for a month, 88% of those with impaired brain blood flow – almost nine out of ten – saw an improvement in blood delivery to brain tissue and better scores on memory and thinking tests.[56]

The cognitive boost they got was not huge (less than ten percent), but allow me to make a couple of observations. First, the benefits were measured after only a month and, second, we older folks should grab for every cognitive boost we can get.

For those whose blood flow was normal at the start of the study, only 37% saw any improvement in blood flow or cognition. The benefits were most obvious among those with the biggest brain health problems at the start.

MRI scans also revealed that those with impaired blood flow were more likely to have small areas of damage to the brain, so maintaining good blood flow is vitally important.

In addition, increasing cerebral blood flow stimulates nerve cell regeneration and even the manufacture of new nerve cells, a process called neurogenesis.

Dr. Farzaneh Sorond, from Harvard Medical School in greater Boston, led the study. She says, "As different areas of the brain need more energy to complete their tasks, they also need greater blood flow. This relationship, called neurovascular coupling, may play an important role in diseases such as Alzheimer's."[57]

This research reinforced earlier findings by Dr. Sorond. In a previous study, 34 healthy people aged 59 to 83 drank two cups of a special, enriched cocoa containing 451 mg of flavanols per cup a day. After one week, blood flow to the brain increased by 8%. After two weeks it increased by 10%.

Improves memory

In another research project, 90 elderly adults with mild cognitive impairment were divided into three groups. Participants in each group drank a cup of cocoa a day containing either 990 mg, 520 mg or 45 mg of flavanols for a period of eight weeks.

At the start of the study they went through a battery of questions and tests for memory,

---

[56] https://www.ncbi.nlm.nih.gov/pubmed/18728792

[57] https://www.ncbi.nlm.nih.gov/pubmed/23925758

attention, language, visual attention, task switching and verbal fluency. This was repeated at the end of the study.

Results showed significant benefits for those taking the medium and high flavanol cocoa. They experienced improvements in short-term, long-term and working memory, processing speed and global cognition. On top of that they enjoyed the benefit of improved insulin resistance, lower blood pressure and decreased free radical activity.[58]

Dr. Giovambattista Desideri, who led the research, commented, "This study provides encouraging evidence that consuming cocoa flavanols….could improve cognitive function."

Reduces damage to nerve pathways

To meticulously study the effects of cocoa, researchers have also used mice specially engineered to develop a disease similar to Alzheimer's.

They looked at the effect of three different extracts of cocoa, with the object of seeing if this food had any effect on the build-up of amyloid plaques. These plaques interfere with gaps between nerve cells (synapses) preventing them from firing properly, disrupting messages and causing damaging inflammation. This process leads to cognitive decline.

The results showed that only a high flavanol extract called Lavano was able to stop the beta amyloid protein from forming sticky lumps.[59]

The study concludes, "Our findings indicate that cocoa extracts have multiple disease-modifying properties in Alzheimer's disease and present a promising route of therapeutic and/or preventative initiatives."

Take the advice of Professor Joe Vinson of the University of Scranton, Pennsylvania, a pioneer in analyzing the health properties of food.

He says cocoa powder has twice as many flavanols as dark chocolate. He recommends making drinks every day using a high flavanol cocoa mix, water or non-fat milk with little or no sugar or a sugar substitute. (P.S. I say avoid the chemical substitutes.)

Restore youth to your brain

Further research now shows chocolate can make your brain effectively *20 to 30 years younger*. That's an astonishing discovery.

The research, led by scientists at the Columbia University Medical Center, indicates you can reverse the decline of a specific section of the brain – one that deteriorates with age – by consuming chocolate. And, in an odd quirk, some researchers believe it's likely that chocolate

---

58 https://www.ncbi.nlm.nih.gov/pubmed/22892813
59 https://www.ncbi.nlm.nih.gov/pubmed/24957018

actually *doesn't* prevent the onset of Alzheimer's. What it does do is prevent or reverse the normal memory loss that comes with age.

During this study, people in their 50s and 60s who consumed a drink containing cocoa flavanols significantly improved their memory skills in the span of just three months.

What goes on in an aging brain

Now, keep in mind that all of us almost inevitably lose some of our intellectual abilities with each passing year. That means that as we reach middle age, we have a harder time remembering names, misplace our car keys more often and spend more time looking for where we parked the car.

For most of us, this gradual memory decline, which usually begins in young adulthood, isn't very noticeable until we reach the age when we're eligible for senior citizen discounts.

Previous studies have suggested, but not proven, that deterioration of an area of the brain called the dentate gyrus causes age-linked brain and memory changes that are not related to Alzheimer's – "normal aging" if you will. So research was designed both to identify changes in the dentate gyrus linked to memory glitches and to see if flavanols from chocolate could help prevent or repair the changes.

The studies reveal good evidence for both of these suppositions.

"When we imaged our research subjects' brains, we found noticeable improvements in the function of the dentate gyrus in those who consumed the high-cocoa-flavanol drink," says researcher Adam M. Brickman.

During this research, people consuming the antioxidants from chocolate took memory tests comparing their memory performance against people who were consuming drinks very low in those antioxidants.

The results of the tests were striking. Chocolate produced HUGE memory improvements.

"If a participant had the memory of a typical 60-year-old at the beginning of the study, after three months that person on average had the memory of a typical 30- or 40-year-old," says researcher Scott A. Small.

Benefits are uneven

As I mentioned, brain scans showed that consuming chocolate increased electrical activity in the dentate gyrus, a part of the larger memory-retaining brain region called the hippocampus. However, activity in another part of the hippocampus called the entorhinal cortex did not increase.

Since the entorhinal cortex suffers serious damage very quickly once you start to experience Alzheimer's, some researchers believe these scanning results point to a novel idea – that normal age-related memory problems are distinct from Alzheimer's damage. In addition, this shows that the flavanols in chocolate may not prevent damage linked to Alzheimer's.

The researchers also point out that most supermarket chocolate candy bars do not contain enough flavanols to produce much help for your brain. You have to eat dark chocolate to derive any benefits. Fortunately, word about the benefits of dark chocolate has gotten out and the stuff is available in all sizes and flavors, from orange to cherry to coconut, at stores that sell healthy food.

Unfortunately, many of these treats still have too much sugar. If you look hard you can find some that are 85% dark chocolate, even 90%, but that's about the highest. (Don't be fooled by ingredients like "dehydrated cane juice." It's sugar, duh.)

I've solved the problem by eating baker's chocolate, which contains no sugar at all. And before you turn up your nose, I have to tell you I've come to like it. As I've said many times, sugar is an addiction and you can wean yourself off it. While I will always love sugar and be tempted by it, I've learned to enjoy food without it.

The studies on chocolate are so convincing, an international group of researchers believe chocolate could potentially be used in "cocoa interventions" to protect young brains from the kind of inflammation – often caused by air pollution – that might otherwise lead to memory problems like Alzheimer's disease.[60]

According to these scientists, "Emerging research suggests that cocoa interventions may be a viable option for neuroprotection, with evidence suggesting that early cocoa interventions could limit the risk of cognitive and developmental concerns."

This is your brain on cocoa

Are these researchers overselling the benefits of chocolate?

If anything, they may not be touting them enough.

Consider research at the University of L'Aquila in Italy. This eight-week study fed hot chocolate to 90 elderly people who were suffering MCI – mild cognitive impairment, the mild memory loss that frequently comes before the development of Alzheimer's disease or other forms of dementia.

The results were undeniable: The seniors' mental performance on cognitive tests improved significantly. What's more, their blood pressure dropped and their insulin resistance was reduced, leading the researchers to note that their better blood sugar control was probably linked to improved mental capacities.

---

60 https://www.ncbi.nlm.nih.gov/pmc/articles/PMC4980563/

Which is not surprising, because an increased risk of brain problems like Alzheimer's has been linked to diabetes and other blood sugar abnormalities.[61] Emerging research has made it clear that diabetes and prediabetes are major causes of dementia. It's quite possible that chocolate's action against high blood sugar is a major cause of its memory benefits.

Add years to your brain's life

Other studies confirm that chocolate should be part of everybody's anti-aging, brain-protection plan. In research called the Maine-Syracuse Longitudinal Study, it has been shown that folks who consume chocolate at least once a week do better on tests of mental function as they get older than do people who never touch chocolate.[62]

As researcher Georgina Crichton explains, the tests used in this study show that eating chocolate can help you do better with daily tasks like "…remembering a phone number, or your shopping list, or being able to do two things at once, like talking and driving at the same time."[63]

In my view, there's no need to wait for further research – a little bit of dark chocolate (which is richest in brain-boosting chemicals) a day may keep your brain problems at bay.

Choline

Choline is emerging as a vital nutrient. Many Americans – perhaps most – suffer from a serious deficiency.

The nutrient is found in some foods and usually classified as being part of the B vitamin group. Although its nutritional importance was discovered in 1932, it was not until 1998 that it was recognized as an essential nutrient by the Food and Nutrition Board of the Institute of Medicine (IOM).

Although the body is able to manufacture choline in the liver, the IOM found that the amount was nowhere near enough to meet human requirements. Along with affecting your brain, choline has critical functions in cell structure, fetal and child development, the cardiovascular system and liver health.

Choline doesn't often occur by itself. It is usually found as a constituent of fats called phosphatidylcholine (PC). These fats form the major structure of cell membranes and make up 30% – nearly a third – of brain tissue. (I hope you're starting to see why choline is so important.) Healthy brain cell membranes are essential to maintain communication between cells. They are vital for cognition, memory, mood and concentration.

---

61   https://www.ncbi.nlm.nih.gov/pubmed/25088942/
62   http://www.sciencedirect.com/science/article/pii/S0195666316300459
63   https://www.washingtonpost.com/news/wonk/wp/2016/03/04/the-magical-thing-eating-chocolate-does-to-your-brain/

PC itself forms part of lecithin, a yellowish-brown fatty substance found in the tissues of animals and plants. Lecithin, PC and choline are often used interchangeably. They're not identical, but, rather like Chinese boxes, lecithin contains PC and PC contains choline.

Although choline has many functions, its most important role is in the brain. In addition to cell membranes, choline is particularly abundant in the mitochondria – the energy factories of all cells, including brain cells – and in the myelin sheaths that surround and protect nerve cells or neurons.

For these reasons the brain has a large appetite for choline, a need that has to be met through either eating certain foods or taking supplements.

Because choline is an important constituent of breast milk, babies have high levels of choline in their blood. This ensures nerve-protective myelin is properly formed and their nervous systems develop normally.

Needed to make a vital neurotransmitter

Perhaps choline's most important role in our bodies is to help produce acetylcholine. This chemical messenger or neurotransmitter is essential for nerve impulses to flow smoothly. This lays the basis for the creation of permanent memories. Choline is one of the few nutritional substances that are able to pass through the blood-brain barrier, enabling the brain to utilize it to make acetylcholine.

Acetylcholine is essential to communication between neurons, including brain cells. It fires up a signal-sending neuron, called a primary neuron, to send its message across the synapse (the gap between the neurons) to stimulate a secondary neuron which receives the signal.

When such a signal is sent and received, the enzyme acetylcholinesterase quickly inactivates acetlycholine. This allows the secondary neuron to rest before being stimulated again. This cycle happens many times per second.

When such impulses occur at a junction between nerve and muscle, the effect is to activate muscle tissue. In other words, acetylcholine is essential to movement and to the nervous system's control and direction of movement.

Unlike other neurotransmitters such as dopamine or serotonin, which are utilized but can be re-uptaken and released again, acetylcholine once inactivated has ended its activity and a fresh supply is needed. Choline is therefore required on a continuous basis.

Choline for a better memory

As we get older a number of changes take place that can lead to memory loss.

Our bodies can produce less acetylcholine or can see an increase in acetylcholinesterase, the enzyme that inactivates acetylcholine. We may experience a loss of cholinergic neurons (nerve cells that produce acetylcholine). Older people may have fewer receptors (molecules that receive chemical signals) for the neurotransmitter to bind to.

We also experience increasing free radical damage as we age, and destruction to parts of the nerve cells themselves, especially the sensitive fatty structures of the dendrites (the branched projections of neurons).

For all these reasons aging causes diminished production of acetylcholine. With this decline, our abilities to think, learn and remember begin to suffer. With this in mind, scientists have been interested to see if supplementing choline can improve acetylcholine levels and, if so, whether the higher levels can improve memory.

When researchers gave healthy volunteers aged 21-29 a single dose of ten grams of choline chloride, their ability to recall unrelated words significantly increased. Those whose memories were poorest at the start of the study were the ones who were helped the most.[64]

Durk Pearson and Sandy Shaw, authors of the best-selling book *Life Extension*, also report that MIT students who took three grams of choline each day had an improved ability to remember a list of words.[65]

1,391 healthy people aged between 36 and 83 filled out a questionnaire about their eating habits, underwent various memory and cognition tests, and also underwent MRI brain scans. The researchers found that those whose diets were high in choline achieved better results on memory tests than did those who consumed little choline.

In addition, the brain scans in this experiment showed those whose diets included the most choline had less white matter hyperintensity (an indicator of diseased blood vessels).

In the medical paper's discussion, the researchers state, "These results support the hypothesis that dietary choline intake is neuroprotective over time and promotes improved cognitive function. We posit that an increase in dietary choline intake ensures adequate acetylcholine concentrations for cholinergic neurotransmission and prevents cell breakdown by preserving phosphatidylcholine within the cell membrane as a result of more choline available to cross the blood-brain barrier."[66]

---

[64] Sitaram et al Choline: Selective enhancement of serial learning and encoding of low imagery words in man Life Sciences Vol. 22 Issue 17 May 1978, 1555–1560

[65] Pearson D & Shaw S. Life Extension, A Practical Scientific Approach. Warner Books 1982

[66] Au R et al The relation of dietary choline to cognitive performance and white-matter hyperintensity in the Framingham Offspring Cohort. American Journal of Clinical Nutrition 2011 Dec;94(6):1584-91

Most bioavailable form of choline

With such important roles in cognition, choline and lecithin have been used experimentally to treat dementia and Alzheimer's disease. However, the results have been mixed. Some early studies showed promise but other researchers were not able to replicate the results.

This has led to the development of other forms of choline that are more bioavailable, i.e. easily utilized by the body.

Citicoline or CDP Choline is a popular form of choline known to be safe, with no side effects. This brain chemical is made naturally by the body and is a precursor to phosphatidylcholine (PC).

Clinical studies have shown Citicoline supports concentration, memory and mental energy. In people who take it, scientists have observed increases in brain levels not only of acetylcholine but also of noradrenaline and dopamine. These neurotransmitters make us feel good, help us focus, improve motivation and raise mental and physical energy.

A review of fourteen human studies found significant beneficial effects of CDP Choline on memory and behavior in chronic cerebral disorders in the elderly.[67]

In a four-week study of 24 elderly people suffering from memory deficits but not dementia, those taking CDP Choline were better able to recall words and objects in memory tests. Researchers stated that "citicoline possesses memory-enhancing activity at doses of 300-1000 mg/day."[68]

Another study involved 95 men and women aged 50 to 85. The researchers concluded that "Citicoline therapy improved verbal memory functioning in older individuals with relatively inefficient memories."[69]

16 healthy volunteers with an average age of 47 participated in a study published in the journal NMR in Biomedicine. People in this group supplemented with CDP Choline for six weeks and received brain scans before and after. The results demonstrated an improvement in brain function. Energy supply to critical brain regions increased by 14%. Test subjects reported feeling sharper, more alert, more productive and more energetic.[70]

---

[67] Fioravanti M, Yanagi M Cytidinediphosphocholine (CDP-choline) for cognitive and behavioural disturbances associated with chronic cerebral disorders in the elderly. Cochrane Database of Systematic Reviews 2005 Apr 18;(2)

[68] Alvarez XA et al Citicoline improves memory performance in elderly subjects. Methods and Findings in Experimental and Clinical Pharmacology 1997 Apr;19(3):201-10.

[69] Spiers PA et al Citicoline improves verbal memory in aging. Archives of Neurology 1996 May;53(5):441-8

[70] Silveri MM et al Citicoline enhances frontal lobe bioenergetics as measured by phosphorus magnetic resonance spectroscopy. NMR in Biomedicine 2008 Nov;21(10):1066-75

GPC used to treat dementia

Another widely-available choline supplement is called choline alfoscerate. It is found naturally in the brain. Choline alfoscerate has shown remarkable results as a treatment for Alzheimer's disease and dementia. However, when taken supplementally by healthy people, insomnia and feelings of being "wired" are common side effects. Most healthy people don't need such a strong form of choline.

In 2003 a Mexican study tested 1200 mg per day of choline alfoscerate, also known as Alpha Glycerol Phosphoryl Choline (Alpha GPC), on 132 patients aged 60 - 80 with mild to moderate Alzheimer's disease. The choline group was compared to 129 patients in a placebo group, using a wide range of tests for cognition.

The researchers found that those taking Alpha GPC saw consistent improvement after 90 and 180 days, whereas those taking the dummy pills either stayed as they were or their condition deteriorated. The researchers concluded, "The results of this study suggest the clinical usefulness and tolerability of choline alfoscerate in the treatment of the cognitive symptoms of dementia disorders of the Alzheimer's type."[71]

These results compare favorably to those obtained from prescription Alzheimer's drugs available as this is written. These drugs pose a number of health risks, and Alpha GPC seems like a reasonable alternative.

A review of ten studies involving dementia patients revealed impressive results with the use of Alpha GPC. These controlled trials included over 1,500 patients with various types of dementia. The review concluded that results in those taking the choline formula were equal to or better than those seen in control groups taking prescribed drugs and superior to those seen in the placebo groups.

The researchers also emphasized that Alpha GPC's ability to relieve cognitive symptoms is what differentiates it from choline and lecithin.[72] The positive results with this formula among dementia patients could be because Alpha GPC also has a number of other roles in brain chemistry beyond being a precursor for acetylcholine.

For example it stimulates the release of another important neurotransmitter called gamma-aminobutyric acid (GABA).[73] Deficiencies of GABA have been linked to Alzheimer's. It also maintains levels of nerve growth factor in the cerebellar cortex, which improves nerve cell communication.[74]

---

71 Moreno DJ, Moreno M. Cognitive improvement in mild to moderate Alzheimer's dementia after treatment with the acetylcholine precursor choline alfoscerate: a multicenter, double-blind, randomized, placebo-controlled trial. Clinical Therapeutics 2003 Jan;25(1):178-93

72 Parnetti L, et al. Choline alphoscerate in cognitive decline and in acute cerebrovascular disease: an analysis of published clinical data. Mech Ageing Dev. 2001 Nov;122(16):2041-55.

73 Ferraro L, et al. Evidence for an in vivo and in vitro modulation of endogenous cortical GABA release by alpha-glycerylphosphorylcholine. Neurochem Res. 1996 May;21(5):547-52.

74 Vega JA, et al. Nerve growth factor receptor immunoreactivity in the cerebellar cortex of aged rats: effect of choline alfoscerate treatment. Mechanism of Ageing and Development. 1993 Jun;69(1-2):119-27

Link to diabetes tested in recent study

Animal research also suggests that choline deficiencies are linked to insulin resistance. This occurs when insulin becomes less able to increase the uptake and utilization of glucose. It often leads to diabetes.

The condition is common in our society, where very high consumption of refined carbohydrates is the norm. When suffering from insulin resistance, our cells simply refuse to take in more glucose – blood sugar; they "resist" insulin, the body's chemical for transporting glucose into our cells. Our cells tell insulin, "We've had enough."

Since there were no human studies on choline and insulin resistance, researchers from Canada enrolled 2,394 men and women over the age of 19 to participate in their study.

The volunteers had their choline and betaine intakes assessed by questionnaire. (Betaine is also found in food and has its own health benefits, but can only be synthesized in the body in the presence of choline).

The researchers also took into account factors that could distort the findings. These were age, sex, calorie intake, physical activity, menopause, smoking, alcohol and medication.

The results were consistent with what was discovered in animals. Those in the top fifth of choline/betaine intake had the lowest insulin resistance. Those with the highest insulin resistance had the lowest choline and betaine intake.[75]

How much should you take?

The IOM set the adequate intake (AI) of choline at 550 milligrams (mg) per day for men and 425 mg per day for women. Choline is found widely in foods, with the best food sources being egg yolks, beef, other meats, liver, salmon, soybeans and wheat germ.

Even so, analysis of dietary intakes found that the average person consumes much less than the recommended dose. Only one person in ten consumes enough choline to meet the required AI.

Conclusion: Most people are deficient in choline.

It was also found that choline intake declines with age, with people aged 71 and older consuming an average of only 264 mg each day. Worse still, recent research has discovered that as much as half the population needs to consume *more* than the IOC's recommendation because of human genetic variations.[76]

---

[75] http://www.nutritionjrnl.com/article/S0899-9007(16)30196-4/fulltext
[76] Zeisel SH, da Costa KA Choline: An Essential Nutrient for Public Health. Nutrition Reviews Nov 2009; 67(11): 615-623

Choline is an overlooked nutrient

It has become clear in recent years that choline is far more important to human health than experts previously thought, because it's involved in vital functions in many systems in the body, particularly the brain. With the incidence of dementia rising sharply, an individual should aim to at least consume the AI – and ideally more.

If it's not possible to achieve this through diet alone, then supplementation is recommended. The evidence available at this time supports the use of Citicoline for healthy people and Alpha GPC for patients diagnosed with Alzheimer's or other forms of dementia.

Cinnamon

According to medical researchers, cinnamon, a simple spice found in most kitchens, could hold the key to defeating Alzheimer's disease.

Tests at the University of California, Santa Barbara, have revealed natural chemicals that appear to slow or completely stop the damaging processes that destroy memory when you get Alzheimer's disease.

Now, you may be familiar with cinnamon's ability to reverse high blood sugar and type 2 diabetes – it's received a lot of publicity. Now it looks like cinnamon may be an answer to dementia, too.

According to the Santa Barbara studies,[77] two chemicals in cinnamon called cinnamaldehyde and epicatechin may prevent the formation of the tangled filaments that clog the brains of Alzheimer's victims.

When you develop Alzheimer's disease, a protein known as tau, which normally plays a key role in building neurons and enabling them to function normally, becomes dysfunctional and starts accumulating in clumps and tangles.

"The problem with tau in Alzheimer's is that it starts aggregating," says researcher Roshni George.

When this protein fails to properly interact with the microtubules that form neuronal structures, it starts to clump together in an unruly mass inside the neurons. As you get older, your brain becomes more vulnerable to developing these sticky masses. And if you develop Alzheimer's, this clumping, entangling phenomenon overwhelms the brain's neurons.

But the California scientists have found that cinnamaldehyde – the compound that gives cinnamon its unforgettable sweet, bright smell – can prevent the formation of tau knots.

---

77 http://www.ncbi.nlm.nih.gov/pubmed/23531502

Apparently, cinnamaldehyde's antioxidant properties stop tau's aggregation (or, in plain English, clumping).

On a molecular scale, cinnamaldehyde forms bonds with two amino acid residues called cysteines that are found on tau protein. By shielding the cysteines, cinnamaldehyde, an oil, prevents the chemical mayhem that promotes Alzheimer's.

Protection from free radicals

"Take, for example, sunburn, a form of oxidative damage," says researcher Donald Graves, Ph.D. "If you wore a hat, you could protect your face and head from the oxidation. In a sense this cinnamaldehyde is like a cap."

Although cinnamaldehyde can shield the tau protein by linking to its cysteine residues, it can also disengage, Dr. Graves says, allowing the correct functions of the protein to proceed.

The natural substance epicatechin, found not only in cinnamon but also in other foods like chocolate, blueberries and red wine, is a powerful antioxidant. Along with preventing cellular damage from those destructive molecules called free radicals, epicatechin is activated by the oxidation process. That enables this chemical to react with the cysteines on the tau protein in a parallel manner to what takes place with cinnamaldehyde.

"Cell membranes that are oxidized also produce reactive derivatives, such as acrolein, that can damage the cysteines," says Roshni George. "Epicatechin also sequesters those byproducts."

If you suffer from type 2 diabetes, you encounter an increased risk of Alzheimer's disease. It is believed that the high blood sugar associated with diabetes results in a large increase in free radicals which are also known as reactive oxygen species. That causes extra oxidative stress. Fortunately, cinnamon can also help in controlling blood sugar.

"Since tau is vulnerable to oxidative stress, this study then asks whether Alzheimer's disease could benefit from cinnamon, especially looking at the potential of small compounds," says Roshni George.

The researchers add that there is still a great deal to learn about cinnamon and its effects on the brain. They warn against taking in large amounts of the substance, though they say that using it in the normal way in cooking is no problem. Our research indicates that one-fourth to one-half teaspoon of cinnamon per day is safe to consume.

It's also a good idea to look for the type of cinnamon that comes from Ceylon and Sri Lanka to keep from consuming coumarin – a blood thinner that occurs in Chinese cinnamon, the type that is most commonly sold in supermarkets. And since cinnamon may kill bacteria, using this spice may have an impact on your intestinal microbes. I haven't seen any studies on that, however.

If eating a half-teaspoon of cinnamon every day is a challenge, you can also take highly potent cinnamon extracts. If you'd like to know more about the best recommended forms of cinnamon – and all about natural ways to beat diabetes – you might want to check out our 241-page book *Defeat High Blood Sugar Naturally!*

"Wouldn't it be interesting if a small molecule from a spice could help?" asks Dr. Graves, "Perhaps prevent it, or slow down the progression?"

Cinnamon targets the hippocampus

Other research, conducted at Rush University in Chicago, shows that ingestion of **cinnamon** may bring about significant changes to the hippocampus – the memory center of the brain – and enhance your learning abilities.[78]

So far, most of the tests and analyses have been performed on rodents. But researcher Kalipada Pahan firmly believes the same effects occur in humans. And what are those effects?

"The increase in learning in poor-learning mice after cinnamon treatment was significant," says Prof. Pahan. He links the boost in learning ability to a chemical the body makes from cinnamon's compounds, sodium benzoate, which is also a preservative used in processed foods.

Now, sodium benzoate may not be a great idea as a food additive because of its interaction with other food ingredients, but when your liver makes this compound from the cinnamon you eat, the chemical crosses the blood-brain barrier and helps neurons regenerate.

The tests at Rush show that the chemical cinnamaldehyde, which endows cinnamon with its unique odor and flavor, is the compound the liver uses to make sodium benzoate.

According to Prof. Pahan, "Sodium benzoate then becomes the active compound, which readily enters the brain and stimulates hippocampal plasticity."

Better learning through cinnamon

In these lab experiments, the researchers found that the hippocampus in the brains of animals that were poor at learning new tasks had an excess of a protein called GABRA5 (Gamma-aminobutyric acid alpha receptor 5). GABRA5 inhibits the transmission of signals between neurons.

At the same time, the slow learners had too little CREB (the acronym for "cAMP response element-binding protein"). CREB has been shown to help with acquiring new knowledge and keeping memories intact over extended periods of time.

Happy news: The consumption of cinnamon fixed both those situations. It raised the amount of memory-boosting CREB and dropped the level of memory-crippling GABRA5.

---

78 http://www.ncbi.nlm.nih.gov/pubmed/27342118

Potential help for Parkinson's disease

In other lab tests at Rush, researchers have found that cinnamon may help change brain malfunctions involved in Parkinson's disease.[79]

These studies showed that the liver's production of sodium benzoate from cinnamon helped ease the movement difficulties that plague Parkinson's sufferers. It also corrected the levels of neurotransmitters that are altered by the disease.

The sodium benzoate increased the supply of the brain proteins known as Parkin and DJ-1, which are sharply lower in the brains of people suffering from Parkinson's disease.

And at least one other test performed on people confirms that sodium benzoate holds promise as a treatment for human memory problems.

This study, performed on about five dozen older folks who were suffering from amnestic mild cognitive impairment and mild Alzheimer's disease, showed that six months of sodium benzoate "substantially improved cognitive and overall functions in patients with early-phase AD (Alzheimer's disease)."[80]

More research is needed, but I expect it's better to help your body manufacture its own sodium benzoate from the foods you eat than it is to ingest this chemical. But – as mentioned earlier – in spite of the potential benefits of cinnamon, don't just go ahead and eat large doses of the spice.

Coconut Oil, MCT Oil

Chances are, you're familiar with the idea of a *ketogenic diet*.

In essence, it means fueling your body with fats instead of carbohydrates. Carbs are metabolized into glucose or blood sugar, which leads to a whole raft of problems from diabetes to cancer to dementia. Fats are an alternate way of providing your body with an energy source, without spiking blood sugar.

A variation on a low-carb diet, the keto diet's main goal is to attain *ketosis*. When you achieve this state, your body is starved for glucose and starts burning fat.

In the phrase that launched a thousand marketing campaigns, the ketogenic diet turns your body into a fat-burning machine.

But please know this... the ketogenic diet is the real deal, not just a fad of weight-loss

---

[79] http://link.springer.com/article/10.1007/s11481-014-9552-2
[80] http://www.ncbi.nlm.nih.gov/pubmed/24074637

enthusiasts and athletes. Researchers into Alzheimer's disease are focusing like a laser beam on carbs as the cause and ketones as one of the solutions.

Ketones offer another source of fuel to brain cells that have lost their ability – thanks to years of abuse – to process glucose.

But there are distinct downsides to trying to go ketogenic...

Not only do you need to completely change the way you eat, but you also need to give your body the time it requires to adjust... which can be uncomfortable.

And for some people, a ketogenic diet is not an option due to health restrictions.[81]

But what if you could get many of the cognitive benefits of ketones while enjoying your usual diet? There is a way.

Coconut oil, MCT oil, and ketones

The benefits of coconut oil are well known, but attention is now being shifted toward MCT oil (medium-chain triglycerides) – one of coconut oil's key nutrients.

In fact, the success of coconut oil in treating Alzheimer's spurred the development of MCT oil, a more concentrated source of the nutrient. This particular fatty acid digests easily, absorbs quickly and is uniquely burned as fuel rather than being stored as fat.

The resulting ketones produced from burning fat can provide energy to a glucose-starved brain.

For many patients with Alzheimer's, insulin resistance has cut off glucose to the brain. But MCTs are a brain food that does not require insulin or glucose to cross the blood-brain barrier. That's why they're able to provide an alternate source of energy to power brain cells.

Are there any risks?

Critics of MCT oil say that adding fats to your diet will only increase your risk of heart disease. This is nonsense. Heart disease is overwhelmingly a product of the high-carb diet, not a diet rich in saturated fats.

A study conducted by the *American Journal of Clinical Nutrition* in 2010 found there was no link between saturated fats (such as the fat found in coconut oil) and heart disease.[82]

Critics also say that unless your diet is fully ketogenic – unless you totally starve yourself of carbs – you will never achieve ketosis and your body will always resort to burning carbohydrates anyway. This is another concern that's unfounded.

---

81 A ketogenic diet for beginners
82 Can MCT Oil Prevent or Reverse Alzheimer's Disease?

In another study published by the journal *Neurobiology of Aging*, patients with Alzheimer's disease or mild cognitive impairment were given either a drink made with MCT oil or a placebo.

In as little as 90 minutes, the MCT-treated group showed significant increases in their levels of ketones. They didn't have to starve themselves of carbs to reap the benefits of MCT oil.[83]

This suggests that the ketones produced from consuming MCT oil are significant enough to afford fuel to the brain even though the diet is not ketogenic.

Dr. Mary Newport pioneered the use of coconut oil and MCT oil for treatment of dementia. Her case studies and investigations make it clear a dementia patient doesn't have to go on a full ketogenic diet to see dramatic improvements in cognition.

She still recommends cutting back on carbs – it's just not necessary to go into full starvation mode. She also recommends combining MCT oil and coconut oil rather than take just one or the other. The MCT oil acts faster but does not last as long. The coconut oil is long-lasting. In a dementia patient, the object is to maintain levels of ketones throughout the day.

If you opt for pure coconut oil, buy the cold-pressed extra virgin form (preferably organic). It can be mixed in with other foods, like oatmeal. For a healthy person seeking to avoid dementia, Dr. Newport recommends three to five tablespoons per day. For someone already in dementia, she recommends four to six tablespoons per day if the patient can tolerate it.

She recommends starting gradually and slowly working up to a higher dose. Some people experience diarrhea or other forms of gastrointestinal distress from taking coconut oil.

In her experience, about half the dementia patients who try coconut oil experience improvement in their symptoms – for instance, they regain the ability to feed themselves or to recognize family members. In some cases the improvements are dramatic.

For more on Dr. Newport's views, see our book *Awakening from Alzheimer's*. She also recommends the best sources of MCT oils (and a variety of other coconut oil products).

---

83 Effects of beta-hydroxybutyrate on cognition in memory-impaired adults.

Curcumin and Turmeric

Since ancient times, turmeric has been called the "spice of life". The people of India consume more of this yellow curry ingredient than anyone else, and have a much lower incidence of Alzheimer's than North Americans and Europeans.

There may be a connection, as scientists uncover more and more evidence of **turmeric's** brain-healthy attributes. Not only can it prevent damage to the brain, it has even been shown to *reverse existing damage*.

The ingredient in turmeric thought responsible for most if not all of its health benefits is called **curcumin**. A curcumin supplement is the easiest way to get a therapeutic dose of turmeric rather than try to eat massive amounts of spicy food.

This view has recently come into question as other curcuminoids found in whole turmeric have been shown to have benefits. But to date, curcumin is the most popular way to reap turmeric's benefits.

A potent antioxidant

Curcumin is a powerful and unique antioxidant, protecting lipids (fats) in brain cell membranes from damage by free radicals. It can do this by a variety of mechanisms. It's able to maintain a high level of activity in important antioxidant enzymes such as catalase, superoxide dismutase (SOD), and glutathione peroxidase.[84]

If you're not an expert on antioxidants, then you might not know that SOD and glutathione are among the most powerful.

It's generally not helpful to take SOD and glutathione as oral supplements because they don't survive passage through the stomach. You need to eat foods that help your body make these antioxidants for itself. So if curcumin is one of those foods, then the yellow spice really is good as gold.

Through its antioxidant action, curcumin also protects the mitochondria – the cell's energy factories – from toxicity. Much of the dysfunction of Alzheimer's is due to mitochondrial damage and outright death. Curcumin can prevent this and enhance the function of these vital cell components.

A powerful anti-inflammatory

Curcumin is also a powerful anti-inflammatory. Inflammation is a feature of Alzheimer's and many other diseases, including cancer, heart disease and arthritis. As Alzheimer's disease

---

[84] http://www.ncbi.nlm.nih.gov/pubmed/17569207

progresses, so does the level of inflammation. Doctors who are successfully treating the disease focus on reducing it.

One study found that taking non-steroidal anti-inflammatory drugs (NSAIDs) for 24 months or more reduced the risk of Alzheimer's dramatically. But these drugs – including familiar names like aspirin and ibuprofen – have serious side effects and cause many deaths each year. A safe anti-inflammatory is urgently needed. Curcumin qualifies.

Curcumin is able to work against many of the steps that lead to inflammation. One example of this is its ability to suppress NF-κB, a protein complex that switches on the inflammatory response.

Helps the Brain Handle Insulin

Blood sugar irregularities create problems with the brain's insulin receptors. Defects in their functioning have been linked with decreased cognitive ability and the development of Alzheimer's.

Several rodent studies have concluded that curcumin's effect on the brain's insulin receptors may be one way it exerts its protective effects against dementia.

Prevents plaques and clears them out

Amyloid plaques that form in the brain are characteristic of Alzheimer's. In fact, these plaques are THE physical mark of Alzheimer's. In animal studies, curcumin has been shown to strike a blow against the disease by preventing these plaques from forming. Many doctors now believe the brain plaques are a response to inflammation, so it makes sense that curcumin would reduce both.

Curcumin is also able to destabilize the plaques even after they've formed. This allows the immune system to clear the amyloid fragments, preventing them from reforming and damaging the brain cells.

Gregory Cole, associate director of the Alzheimer's Disease Center at the University of California at Los Angeles, is very enthusiastic about the potential of curcumin. Commenting on one study he said, "In one week, curcumin reduced the average size of the plaques by 30 percent. They could see the plaques disappearing.

"The prospect of finding a safe and effective approach to both prevention and treatment of Alzheimer's disease is tremendously exciting. There's real potential for curcumin in treating brain diseases."

Along with these benefits, researchers at the University of Michigan have found the curcumin may help prevent Parkinson's disease by keeping proteins from misfolding and clumping together – misfolded, aggregated proteins can cause the type of neuron damage that leads to Parkinson's.[85]

It appears your health can benefit from even moderate consumption of curcumin-rich turmeric.[86]

Dr. Tze-Pin Ng, from the National University of Singapore, said that it is remarkable, but his research suggests a person needs to consume curry just once in a while to see a positive effect on mental health.

However, other evidence I've seen suggests that the larger the dose, the more effective. I know of at least one doctor who is using enormous doses of curcumin intravenously on patients with advanced disease.

I take a curcumin supplement every day myself. I won't call this habit a "no-brainer." It's a "have-more-brainer"!

Vitamin D

Vitamin D is so important for preserving brain health, if it were a drug, pharmaceutical companies would charge you a small fortune to buy it at your local pharmacy.

It cuts your risk of dementia and memory loss in old age in half. And that's just for starters…

If you suffer cardiac arrest, cutting off blood flow, this vitamin improves your chances of retaining good brain function sevenfold. (Oh, and while we're on the subject, it also boosts your chance of surviving the heart attack.)

The vitamin also increases brain power in middle age.

Almost everyone is deficient

Despite this vitamin's importance, experts estimate that 70 percent of us aren't getting enough. I would say the 70 percent figure is conservative. In a moment, I'm going to share with you some shocking news about how much vitamin D you *should* be taking, and I guarantee you that even good alternative doctors are NOT up to speed on the latest research.

First, let's look at the incredible benefits those high vitamin D levels can give you…

Researchers at the University of Exeter Medical School in the United Kingdom conducted

---

85 https://www.ncbi.nlm.nih.gov/pubmed/22267729
86 https://www.ncbi.nlm.nih.gov/pubmed/16870699

an international study.[87] The results show that if you enter old age with a significant vitamin D deficiency you run a doubled risk of dementia and Alzheimer's disease compared to people who have adequate amounts of the vitamin.

The scientists analyzed data from senior Americans who were taking part in research called the Cardiovascular Health Study. People in the study who were only moderately vitamin D deficient ran a 53 percent increased risk of developing dementia of any sort as they aged. The people who were severely lacking in vitamin D were at 125 percent greater risk – far more than a double.

Parallel findings were found for Alzheimer's disease: People who were moderately deficient were 69 percent more vulnerable to this type of memory problem, and the risk of the severely deficient grew by 122 percent.

According to researcher David Llewellyn, "We expected to find an association between low Vitamin D levels and the risk of dementia and Alzheimer's disease, but the results were surprising – we actually found that the association was twice as strong as we anticipated."

Protect your heart and brain

Researchers in South Korea looked into the effects of vitamin D on people who suffer cardiac arrest (when the heart's steady rhythm is interrupted and the heart has to be restarted). The study found an even more impressive level of protection.[88]

Cardiac arrest interrupts the blood supply to the brain, threatening the survival of brain cells. But having sufficient vitamin D exerted strong protection against disruption of brain cell function. "Vitamin D deficiency increased the risk of poor neurological outcome after sudden cardiac arrest by sevenfold," notes researcher Wi Jin.

He also reports that six months after their cardiac arrests, a third of the vitamin D deficient patients had died. None of the people who had enough vitamin D in their bodies passed away during that time.

Better cognition

Meanwhile, if you're trying to improve your brain power in middle age, research at the University of Manchester in England shows that higher levels of vitamin D improve your intellectual abilities. This study[89] looked at how well more than 3,300 European men in their 40s, 50s, 60s and 70s performed on tests of their mental focus and processing of information.

---

87 http://www.ncbi.nlm.nih.gov/pubmed/25098535
88 http://www.escardio.org/about/press/press-releases/pr-14/Pages/vitamin-D-deficiency-impacts-brain-function.aspx (Reference accessed at time of original publication; may no longer be available)
89 http://www.ncbi.nlm.nih.gov/pubmed/19460797

"Interestingly, the association between increased vitamin D and faster information processing was more significant in men aged over 60 years, although the biological reasons for this remain unclear," reports researcher David Lee. "The positive effects vitamin D appears to have on the brain need to be explored further but certainly raise questions about its potential benefit for minimizing aging-related declines in cognitive performance."

Influences the neurotransmitter of happiness

Vitamin D may also help keep you from getting depression by improving the balance of serotonin in your brain, a neurotransmitter associated with good mood and feelings of wellbeing.

The research on vitamin D and depression makes it clear that much of the proliferation of this mental condition may be the result of bad advice from doctors.

Think about what doctors often give people who are depressed – drugs called selective serotonin reuptake inhibitors (SSRIs). These include drugs like Prozac, Paxil, Zoloft, Celexa and Lexapro.

SSRIs are supposed to help the brain retain more serotonin and thereby keep your mood upbeat. But meanwhile, another group of doctors is undermining your SSRI levels.

While one group of doctors hands out pills right and left to boost SSRI levels, other practitioners – dermatologists – are telling people to stay out of the sun to keep the skin from tanning and burning.

How are those two facts related? Researchers now know that missing out on the vitamin D your skin makes from the sun can lead to depression in many people. Not only that – the body uses vitamin D to produce serotonin, the very neurotransmitter that medical folks often think we lack!

You can see what I'm getting at – If more people got more vitamin D from sunlight, there might be fewer depressed people who think they need to take antidepressant drugs.

It looks like medical research is starting to catch up with this paradox. A study at Oregon State University has demonstrated that low levels of vitamin D in the body are linked to an increased risk of depression in women who are otherwise healthy.

The study looked at young women who live in the Pacific Northwest who have a big risk for depression. As it happens, they also live in a part of the country that is notorious for its cloudy, dreary weather. During the winter months, what little sunshine there is in this region isn't strong enough to stimulate much vitamin D production in the body.[90]

Researcher David Kerr, a Ph.D. and Associate Professor at Oregon State, observes that "Depression has multiple, powerful causes and if vitamin D is part of the picture, it is just a small

---

[90] http://www.ncbi.nlm.nih.gov/pubmed/25791903

part. But given how many people are affected by depression, any little inroad we can find could have an important impact on public health."

How your body makes serotonin

Meanwhile, a study at the Children's Hospital Oakland Research Institute has unraveled the intricate relationship among vitamin D, omega-3 fats (such as those found in fish oil) and the brain's production of serotonin.[91]

This research shows that vitamin D is crucial for serotonin production – it controls the body's conversion of the essential amino acid tryptophan into serotonin.

Omega-3s help with serotonin by stimulating its release from one set of the brain's neurons and then easing serotonin's passage into other neurons that need it to function properly. The Oakland scientists note that we are not getting enough vitamin D or omega-3s to keep our brains healthy.

"Vitamin D, which is converted to a steroid hormone that controls about 1,000 genes, many in the brain, is a major deficiency in the US and omega-3 fatty acid deficiencies are very common because people don't eat enough fish," says researcher Bruce Ames.

And you can't argue with the Oregon researchers who think that even if vitamin D supplements aren't a miracle cure, more people should take them. "Vitamin D supplements are inexpensive and readily available," says Dr. Kerr. "They certainly shouldn't be considered as alternatives to the treatments known to be effective for depression, but they are good for overall health."

At the same time, a flurry of examinations of the brain's structure and function have long suggested that the brain can't keep going for very long without vitamin D.

The brain is chock full of receptors for vitamin D, consisting of molecular structures designed to grab on to the nutrient and put it to use. In particular, the cells of the hippocampus – the part of the brain responsible for preserving many of our memories – is dense with vitamin D receptors.

These brain cells are also rich in 1alpha-hydroxylase, an enzyme that converts circulating vitamin D into a form that can enter the cells and be active.[92]

Plus, lab tests have shown that vitamin D helps keep the brain clear of amyloid plaque, the sticky clumps of destructive protein that can accumulate there and cause the neuron disruption linked to Alzheimer's disease. Vitamin D increases the activity of macrophages, immune cells that literally eat these problematic proteins.[93]

---

91 http://www.ncbi.nlm.nih.gov/pubmed/25713056
92 http://www.ncbi.nlm.nih.gov/pubmed/15589699
93 http://www.med.upenn.edu/shorterlab/Papers/Member%20Papers/fulltext.pdf

In addition, studies show that vitamin D can keep your brain larger as you age and prevent it from atrophying[94] – i.e. shrinking. And it doesn't stop there. Vitamin D lowers the risk of strokes and circulation problems in brain tissue.[95] Brain shrinkage is natural with age, but you want to do everything you can to slow it down – and vitamin D is one of the ways.

Grow new brain tissue

Meanwhile, other studies show that vitamin D can help regenerate axons in the brain. Axons are projections from the neurons that transmit impulses in the brain.[96] They are bundled together and form important paths for sending signals from one cell to the next. Some researchers believe that vitamin D will someday be used in therapies to repair the axons in damaged spinal columns.[97]

From across the Atlantic comes confirmation of the stats I quoted at the beginning of this article showing massive increases in dementia among people who don't have enough D. At the University of Exeter in England, a six-year study of seniors demonstrated that moderate deficiency in vitamin D ups your risk of Alzheimer's disease by almost 70 percent.

Their analysis also indicated that if you have a severe D deficiency, your risk jumps more than 120 percent, compared to people who have sufficient levels of this nutrient.[98]

The research looked at the brain health of more than 1,650 people over the age of 65. They found that to protect your brain, your blood test for 25(OH)D – a measure of your vitamin D status – should be at or over 50 nmol/L.

Although no one has pinpointed the optimal dose of vitamin D,[99] taking supplements obviously seems to be a good preventive measure for keeping your brain healthy. Few other nutrients are as important for brain power.

How much D is enough?

You probably need far more vitamin D than you ever thought, and far more than even ardent alternative doctors are likely to recommend.

For years, mainstream medical authorities stupidly and ignorantly told the public it was dangerous to take more than 400 IU a day. As recently as eight years ago the medical authorities were attacking doctors who suggested that far more vitamin D was needed and that supplements of 2000 IU per day were safe for most adults.

---

94 http://www.ncbi.nlm.nih.gov/pubmed/23281306
95 http://www.ncbi.nlm.nih.gov/pubmed/23225498
96 http://www.ncbi.nlm.nih.gov/pubmed/18986226
97 http://www.ncbi.nlm.nih.gov/pubmed/24948020
98 http://www.neurology.org/content/early/2014/08/06/WNL.0000000000000755.short
99 http://annals.org/article.aspx?articleid=1938935

As evidence has piled up, mainstream medicine has backed off and now acknowledges some of the amazing benefits of vitamin D, but they're still far behind the best science on this subject. If you believe what your conventional, mainstream doctor tells you about vitamin D, you are putting your health at serious risk.

Vitamin D is well tolerated at doses of up to 2,000 IU daily for adults. But the truth is, even 2000 is too timid and conservative. There is almost no danger of toxicity – and abundant evidence of huge benefits to your health – at much higher doses.

Many studies suggest we should aim for 35 IU's per pound of body weight. That would put the daily requirement at more than 5,000 IU for a person who weighs 150 pounds. Sunshine on exposed skin is the best source, when weather and time of year permit.

A blood test is the only way to ensure your vitamin D levels are adequate and to help you adjust your supplement intake to make sure you're getting what you need. You may be in for a surprise. Despite taking 4,000 to 5,000 IU of vitamin D per day and getting quite a bit of sun as well, I recently found that my own blood levels were still too low according to a blood test.

By dint of taking 10,000 IUs per day for about a year, I finally got my blood level to 53. I want to see it go above 60. And stay there.

If you get yourself tested, here's what the numbers mean

The blood test measures your vitamin D levels in terms of nanograms of vitamin C per deciliter of blood. You want your level to be above 60, and my research team has learned from interviews conducted with top doctors that, in fact, blood levels as high as 60 are rare. Blue moons occur far more often than patients who have D levels above 60.

In other words, nearly everyone is deficient.

If you've got a serious disease of aging like cancer or Alzheimer's, levels of 80 to 100 are desirable, some doctors say. (I hasten to add this is not widely accepted.) Such levels are nearly unheard of.

When I set out to get my blood level above 60, I started at 40 – and I had been supplementing with 4,000 – 5,000 IU of vitamin D per day for a long time! I then upped it to ten per twelve thousand per day.

What about toxicity? Excessive levels of vitamin D can lead to excessive levels of calcium in the blood, which can be toxic. I'm not aware of large studies on the subject, but in an interview one doctor told us that a D level of about 160 appeared to be the danger point. Readings that high are so rare, it's unlikely a doctor who has tested hundreds of patients has ever seen a patient with a toxic vitamin D level.

Muscle spasms are a symptom of the toxic condition, and if you suddenly start experiencing those after a long period supplementing with large amounts of vitamin D, it would be wise to cut back on the vitamin and get yourself tested again. The ideal way to supplement with vitamin D is under the guidance of an informed doctor who knows what he's doing. That's what I recommend. There is no way to know how much you need without periodic blood testing.

Vitamin E

Vitamins are good for you, right? Then how come so many health "experts" keep raising doubts about the safety of vitamin E? Amping up the fear are published, peer-reviewed studies that seem to show taking vitamin E may hasten your demise and increase your risk of diseases like cancer.

But don't be too hasty to give up on vitamin E supplements – much less avoid E-rich foods like spinach, avocado or walnuts. If you truly understand this nutrient, you'll realize it can help keep your brain functioning well into old age.

One complicating factor in this scientific analysis is that not everything labeled vitamin E is the same substance. At least eight different forms of vitamin E are found in nature, and adding to the confusion are synthesized, i.e. manufactured varieties. Some of these varieties may be useless for health. But other forms help protect your health and brain function. But you have to know which is which.

Maret Traber is a Principal Investigator at the Linus Pauling Institute and a full professor at Oregon State University. She's performed intense research on all the forms of vitamin E, and holds that worries about vitamin E are unfounded because so-called "experts" who claim to have uncovered indications that vitamin E supplements can lead to things like cancer are not analyzing the research results correctly.[100]

"I believe that past studies which have alleged adverse consequences from vitamin E have misinterpreted the data," she says. "Taking too much vitamin E is not the real concern. A much more important issue is that more than 90 percent of people in the US have inadequate levels of vitamin E in their diet."

She points out that vitamin E acts as a fat-soluble antioxidant that protects virtually all the cell membranes in the body. It also operates as an anticoagulant that prevents excessive blood clotting. And 90 percent of all Americans don't get enough vitamin E.

---

100 https://www.ncbi.nlm.nih.gov/pmc/articles/PMC3735929/

Vitamin E gets nutrients into the brain

One of vitamin E's functions is to help move brain-protecting nutrients into the brain.

For instance, although many people know that the brain depends on omega-3 fatty acids – the type of fats found in fish oil – to stay healthy and keep their memories working, not many know that vitamin E is necessary for getting omega-3s into the brain where they can help keep neurons healthy.

The body uses omega-3 fats to create protective brain cell membranes that keep neurons from being damaged. This is crucial for having a better brain as you age, because when these membranes are compromised, your neurons become much more vulnerable to memory-destroying problems like Alzheimer's disease.

Your body can't make omega fatty acids for itself. You have to take them in from your food. When you consume these fats in your diet, they are first sent to the liver, which turns them into a form that can be sent to the brain and absorbed.

"(Our) research showed that vitamin E is needed to prevent a dramatic loss of a critically important molecule in the brain, and helps explain why vitamin E is needed for brain health," says Prof. Traber. "Human brains are very enriched in DHA [one of the omega-3s] but they can't make it, they get it from the liver."

The evidence leaves little doubt

Prof. Traber's lab research has focused on the brain-protective role of docosahexaenoic acid (DHA), the most important omega-3 fat. DHA is part of a substance called DHA-PC that is incorporated into the membranes of every brain cell.

Her research shows that a vitamin E deficiency can lead to a 30 percent lower level of DHA-PC in the brain.

That's dangerous: Other researchers have found that when you have less DHA-PC circulating in your body (much of it on the way to your brain), you run a much higher risk of Alzheimer's disease.

To get to the brain, DHA-PC is transported in compounds called lyso-pls. They allow the DHA-PC to cross the blood-brain barrier and be used as a building block for repairing brain cell membranes.

Deficiency problem

In Prof. Traber's tests, a deficiency in vitamin E was associated, on average, with a whopping 60 percent drop-off in lyso-pls.

"The particular molecules that help carry (DHA to the brain) are these lyso-pls, and the amount of those compounds is being greatly reduced when vitamin E intake is insufficient," warns Dr. Traber. "This sets the stage for cellular membrane damage and neuronal death."

As Prof. Traber points out, other studies have shown that people suffering the early stages of Alzheimer's can be helped somewhat by taking vitamin E. But by the time Alzheimer's has started, she says, years of neurological damage have already taken place that cannot be reversed by merely supplementing with vitamin E.

"You can't build a house without the necessary materials," Dr. Traber warns. "In a sense, if vitamin E is inadequate, we're cutting by more than half the amount of materials with which we can build and maintain the brain."

Buy natural, avoid synthetic

Another issue with vitamin E is the fact that there exists both a natural form and a manufactured variety. The body is much more efficient at using the natural form. Most of the synthetic form is physiologically useless. On supplement packages, synthetic forms of vitamin E are generally denoted as dl-tocopherols, while the more desirable natural forms are the d-tocopherols.

The eight natural forms of vitamin E consist of four tocopherols, each with a different role in the body, plus four more substances called tocotrienols. Each comes in four forms, denoted Alpha, Beta, Delta and Gamma. Thus there is an "alpha tocopherol" and an "alpha tocotrienol" and likewise for Beta, Delta and Gamma.

Knowledgeable vitamin E researchers point out that studies that show no benefit to vitamin E almost always focus on synthetic vitamin E or involve people who only take alpha tocopherol, not the other seven forms of vitamin E. The tocotrienol forms are, in fact, hard to find and only knowledgeable people take them.

When researchers take into account all forms of Vitamin E, their results actually turn up significant health benefits.

For example, a Swedish study found that older people who have high levels of several forms of vitamin E circulating in their blood enjoy a lower risk for Alzheimer's disease.[101]

As research leader Francesca Mangialasche, M.D., points out, "Vitamin E is a family of eight natural components, but most studies related to Alzheimer's disease investigate only one of these components, alpha tocopherol.

We hypothesized that all the vitamin E family members could be important in protecting against AD [Alzheimer's disease]. If confirmed, this result has implications for both individuals and society, as 70 percent of all dementia cases in the general population occur in people over

---

[101] http://www.ncbi.nlm.nih.gov/pubmed/20413888

75 years of age, and the study suggests a protective effect of vitamin E against AD in individuals aged 80+."

The Swedish study examined blood samples from 232 people over the age of 80 who were clear-minded at the start of the research. Six years later, the scientists found that 57 of the participants had developed Alzheimer's disease.

When the researchers looked at levels of the eight natural vitamin E components in the blood samples taken at the initial stage of the study, they found that the people who had the highest level of various forms of the vitamin enjoyed a reduced risk of Alzheimer's of up to 54 percent. Their risk of Alzheimer's was less than half that of the people with low levels.

Combine the various forms of E

Dr. Mangialasche points out that vitamin E's protective effect appears to be linked to the combination of the various forms of the vitamin.

"Elderly people as a group are large consumers of vitamin E supplements, which usually contain only alpha tocopherol, and this often at high doses", says Dr. Mangialasche. "Our findings need to be confirmed by other studies, but they open up the possibility that the balanced presence of different vitamin E forms can have an important neuroprotective effect."

If you take vitamin E, make sure you take a supplement that has natural E and includes a mixture of the various forms. That offers your best bet for brain and health protection.

The research I've seen suggests that the four tocotrienols are the most powerful and effective forms of vitamin E – NOT the four tocopherols. Unfortunately, tocotrienol supplements tend to be expensive and harder to find. But I make sure I take a tocotrienol supplement every other day. On the alternate days, I take a supplement that contains a mixture of all four tocopherols.

Prof. Traber notes that vitamin E in food is usually supplied by cooking oils like olive oil. But many people don't eat the foods richest in vitamin E – things like avocados, almonds and sunflower seeds.

If you take vitamin E supplements, take *natural* vitamin E made up of mixed tocopherols and tocotrienols. These high-quality vitamin E supplements comprised of multiple forms of E are more than worth the trouble and extra cost.

The body is not able to effectively put synthetic vitamin E to good use. Most common vitamin E supplements contain only alpha tocopherol, which is not very nutritious by itself, and may even be harmful, according to some studies, if not taken in combination with the other forms of vitamin E.

Low vitamin E means poorer memory

Studies of older people confirm vitamin E's importance. They indicate that seniors who are very low in vitamin E run a greater risk of experiencing memory difficulties.

Research in Finland, for instance, that measured the blood levels of vitamin E in people over age 65 shows that the types of vitamin E known as gamma-tocopherol and beta-tocotrienol are most important for a better memory as are the total tocotrienol levels in people's blood.[102]

To get more vitamin E in your meals and snacks, eat foods relatively rich in vitamin E like sunflower seeds, almonds, spinach, avocado and red pepper.

Ecklonia cava

In the late 1980s and early 1990s, three PhD students at the University of Iowa were developing drugs to combat cardiovascular disease and Alzheimer's disease.

They started to question the conventional tactic, which was to focus on inhibiting certain biochemical responses. Blocking biochemical processes often comes with unwanted – and sometimes deadly – side effects.

So they switched gears and focused on finding ways to boost the body's natural defense mechanisms. After years of research they discovered that elements in seaweed and algae are powerful antioxidants that can reduce the risk of developing dementia and Alzheimer's disease.

These superior compounds come from *Ecklonia cava*, a red-brown seaweed that grows at least 100 feet under the sea off the coasts of Japan and South Korea.

The beneficial chemicals in Ecklonia cava are unique polyphenols and phlorotannins (tannins specific to red-brown seaweed). These polyphenols are also considered flavonoids, antioxidants and anti-inflammatories.

What makes Ecklonia cava so effective?

The polyphenols in Ecklonia are different from those extracted from land sources.

Antioxidants get their free-radical fighting power from their molecular structure, which is made of interconnected rings. The rings are what capture stray electrons and restore balance to free-radical-damaged cells. The more rings an antioxidant has, the more effective it is.

Most land-sourced polyphenols have two or three rings. Green tea catechins, considered one of the most potent antioxidants in the world, have four rings.

---

102 http://www.sciencedirect.com/science/article/pii/S0531556513002878?via%3Dihub

Ecklonia cava has eight interconnected rings. Having twice as many rings as any other antioxidant makes *Ecklonia cava* 10-100 times more effective than land-based polyphenols.

It also lasts longer. Most land-based polyphenols are water soluble and have a 30-minute half-life. This isn't surprising, considering the human body is between 57-60% water.[103]

But *Ecklonia cava* is 40% lipid (fat) soluble. Its half-life is as much as 12 hours. Because it breaks down more slowly in the body, it's much more effective.

Being fat soluble also means it can cross the blood-brain barrier (BBB for short – a kind of biological "firewall" that protects the brain). Once inside the brain, the ingredients in the formula protect neurons from oxidative damage and death. The formula can also penetrate all the cells in the body more effectively than water soluble compounds.

Ecklonia cava boosts the brain in animal studies

In addition to combatting oxidative damage – and reducing associated inflammation – in the brain and neurons, the antioxidants in *Ecklonia cava* **effectively combat peroxynitrites**, a specific class of free radicals that are toxic to neurons.[104]

Peroxynitrites interact with lipids, DNA and proteins in the body and brain. They cause "overwhelming oxidative injury, committing [healthy] cells to necrosis or apoptosis." These free radicals can also trigger strokes, chronic inflammatory diseases and neurodegenerative disorders.[105]

In animal studies, *Ecklonia cava* increased the memory-related neurotransmitter acetylcholine by 140% in brain regions responsible for learning and memory.[106] If you read the choline chapter in this book you know that acetylcholine is essential to a healthy brain.

Low levels of acetylcholine are associated with an increased amount of beta amyloid plaques and Alzheimer's disease. Researchers have eagerly searched for ways to stimulate the production of this essential neurotransmitter as a possible preventative measure for mild cognitive impairment (MCI) and dementia.

Another study in rats showed those that received *Ecklonia cava* performed better in a water maze than did the control group, suggesting that this seaweed supplement can improve short term memory.[107] . (It's also important to note that these animal studies are not the last word. Human studies are needed for confirmation.)

---

103 How much of your body is water?

104 *The Encyclopedia of Medical Breakthroughs and Forbidden Treatments*. Published by Medical Research Associates, Seattle, WA.

105 Nitric oxide and peroxynitrite in health and disease.

106 *The Encyclopedia of Medical Breakthroughs and Forbidden Treatments*. Published by Medical Research Associates, Seattle, WA.

107 Lee, B. Unpublished research, Hanbat National University, Korea. National Institute of Aging, National Institutes of Health, 2004.

A study of lab-cultured cells, published in the *Journal of the Korean Society of Food Science and Nutrition*, compared the antioxidant levels of various kinds of seaweed and found that *Ecklonia cava* had the highest total polyphenol content out of 20 varieties.

The researchers found *Ecklonia cava* reduced neuron death, reduced the levels of beta-secretase (one of the enzymes that create amyloid plaque) and increased acetylcholine.

They concluded, "*Ecklonia cava* extract has potential anti-dementia activity, which suggests that it might provide an effective strategy for improving dementia."[108]

And finally, a study published in the journal *NeuroToxicology* concluded that the phlorotannins in *Ecklonia cava* can reduce beta-amyloid plaque production by inhibiting amyloid precursor protein (APP), gamma-secretase and alpha-secretase.[109]

Best ways to get Ecklonia cava into your daily routine

While seaweed provides a rich menu of nutrients, the polyphenols are not very concentrated. You'd have to eat a great deal of it to get the benefits I've described. Assuming you can find a place to purchase it.

You'd be better off supplementing with up to 720 mg of an *Ecklonia cava supplement* daily. It's available in a branded ingredient called Seanol. Many products go by different names and say "with Seanol" somewhere on the label. Just be aware that so far the proof of the benefits appears to be animal studies (unless there are human studies I'm not aware of.) Animal studies are not conclusive for human benefits.

Fisetin

The chemical compound **fisetin**, found most abundantly in **strawberries**, possesses the power to ward off multiple diseases – particularly inflammatory diseases affecting the brain, like Alzheimer's.

Early research is so promising, it may turn out to be a nutritional miracle. Besides being a possible dementia treatment, it's an anti-carcinogen – and a calming agent to boot.

Scientists from the Salk Institute for Biological Studies have found that fisetin, when fed to genetically altered mice, *completely eliminates Alzheimer's symptoms* and prevents the disease from destroying natural brain function.[110]

---

108 In vitro screening for anti-dementia activities of seaweed extracts.
109 Phlorotannin-rich Ecklonia cava reduces the production of beta-amyloid by modulating alpha- and gamma-secretase expression and activity.
110 http://www.ncbi.nlm.nih.gov/pubmed/24341874

Their experiments showed that fisetin automatically targets a protein known as p35, which causes inflammation and degeneration of brain tissue. Fisetin helped reverse p35's pathway, allowing the brain to function normally.

The substance also increased memory capacity in the mice.

Most significantly, it did all this *without touching* the amyloid beta plaques and tau tangles characteristic of Alzheimer's disease.

This is very important, so it's worth repeating:

Normal brain function means no symptoms, even when plaques were present and the disease continued to progress.[111]

If the findings hold up in human studies (and there's already some indication they will) this could be an important development.

The fact that *symptoms* are treatable without targeting the plaques is very exciting. Major drug company researchers have mainly focused on curing plaque build-up. The strategy has not been successful and the drugs have failed. Many leading Alzheimer's experts now believe the whole "plaque theory of Alzheimer's disease" is mistaken.

Now, the new fisetin research seems to support that view. Fisetin reversed the symptoms of Alzheimer's without affecting plaque. If it does likewise in human patients, they'll be able to live longer, while leading more enjoyable lives.

This discovery should change the priorities of future research entirely.

High levels of fisetin are found in other fruits and vegetables besides strawberries:

- Blueberries
- Mangoes
- Apples
- Persimmon
- Kiwi
- Grapes
- Onions
- Cucumber

According to the Alzheimer's Research & Prevention Foundation, eating at least nine servings of colorful fruits and vegetables daily will help protect memory.[112]

---

111 http://www.liveinthenow.com/article/rare-compound-in-strawberries-may-curb-alzheimers-disease
112 Fisetin: A natural compound that fights memory loss.

The skins of these foods contain the most fisetin. To get the most nutritional impact, eat them raw with the skins.

If they must be cooked, then steaming or cooking slowly at temperatures below 200 degrees will help keep the nutrients intact. Rapid boiling and cooking at high heat will destroy fisetin compounds and other delicate nutrients.

If you plan to eat the skins of fruits and vegetables, your best bet is to buy organic, especially when the food you're buying is on the Environmental Working Group's (EWG) Dirty Dozen list. This is a list of the foods most contaminated by chemical and industrial pesticides, when grown the conventional way. Strawberries, apples and grapes are all on the list.[113]

Berry, berry good!

But experts have estimated you'd have to eat approximately 37 strawberries per day to match the amount of fisetin used in the animal studies.

That's about a pound and a half of medium sized berries. It might seem like a lot ...

But one collaborative study conducted by the University of Granada and the Marche Polytechnic University gave 1.1 pounds to participants daily for two weeks.

The only "side effects" were increased antioxidant capacity of the blood and resistance to cell fragmentation (which can cause a number of serious diseases.)[114]

The finding was confirmed by the University of Warwick, which showed that strawberries positively activate a protein called Nrf2, which decreases cholesterol levels and protects the cardiovascular system from disease.[115]

What's more, strawberries have also been found to help balance blood sugar after you eat, reducing the risk of diabetes (and helping fight it for those who already have the disease). People with diabetes are at much higher risk for developing Alzheimer's later in life. (Alzheimer's is often referred to as "type 3 diabetes" because it's associated with high blood sugar.) It's not surprising that a remedy for one of these diseases is a remedy for the other, too.

The bottom line

I can confidently recommend making fresh, organic strawberries a regular part of your diet. Enjoying a handful with every meal and as a snack could have powerful benefits.

If you'd like to achieve a clinical dose, eating such a large quantity of strawberries daily sounds like a tall order. Fortunately, fisetin supplements are available.

---

113 Dirty Dozen.
114 www.sciencedaily.com/releases/2011/06/110621074314.htm
115 www.sciencedaily.com/releases/2012/07/120704124107.htm

As always, do what feels right to you and confirm everything with your doctor.

Fish Oil

If you don't consume fish oil every day, most experts agree you're experiencing a "nutrition gap" that omits a powerful brain-boosting nutrient that is woefully low in our diets.[116] In fact, fish oil may be the most frequently recommended food or supplement for brain health.

That's because it has the potential to protect you against Alzheimer's disease and keep your brain from shrinking as you age – as well as producing a host of other health benefits (better cardiovascular health, for example).

Brain shrinkage is a so-called "natural" result of aging, but it's accelerated by poor diet and other health habits. This nutrient can help slow it down or stop it.

The key to fish oil's benefits are its **omega-3 fatty acids** – DHA (docosahexaenoic acid) and EPA (eicosapentaenoic acid).

Eat this, get a bigger brain

Researchers in a six month study gave daily doses of DHA to a group of older adults who were already suffering MCI – mild cognitive impairment, meaning their memories were starting to slip. The scientists found that it improved the patients' memory and learning abilities.[117]

According to Duff MacKay, a naturopathic doctor with the Council for Responsible Nutrition, "The results of this study are very encouraging for those consumers concerned about maintaining memory. We know that lower DHA levels are associated with cognitive decline in healthy elderly and Alzheimer's patients, and higher DHA levels help reduce the risk of Alzheimer's disease."

Even though this research showed that fish oil could help those who were already having memory difficulties, Dr. MacKay and others believe that **the sooner you start consuming nutrients like DHA and EPA, the better**.

More evidence for fish oil

A study of more than a thousand women in their late 70s showed that those who had higher levels of omega-3 fatty acids in their blood had larger brains. That kind of increased brain size reduces your risk of Alzheimer's disease. It's a remarkable finding – a **higher DHA level equals a bigger brain**.[118]

---

116 http://www.ift.org/newsroom/news-releases/2013/july/16/nutrition-gap-in-omega-3-fatty-acids.aspx
117 http://www.ift.org/newsroom/news-releases/2013/july/16/nutrition-gap-in-omega-3-fatty-acids.aspx
118 http://www.ift.org/newsroom/news-releases/2013/july/16/nutrition-gap-in-omega-3-fatty-acids.aspx

"These higher levels of fatty acids can be achieved through diet and the use of supplements, and the results suggest that the effect on brain volume is the equivalent of delaying the normal loss of brain cells that comes with aging by one to two years," says researcher James V. Pottala, Ph.D., of the University of South Dakota.

In Dr. Pottala's research, the women with more EPA and DHA in their blood had brains whose hippocampus was 2.7 percent larger. The hippocampus is a key brain structure when it comes to the memory function. People doomed to Alzheimer's experience a shrinking hippocampus even before their memories start to degrade. A size boost of 2.7 percent may not sound like much, but it's highly significant.

Early brain protection

Research on lab animals supports the benefit of beginning to consume EPA and DHA *before* your mental capacity begins to slip. In one of these studies, when animals that had been genetically altered to develop Alzheimer's began an EPA-enriched diet early in life (along with receiving B vitamins and other nutrients) their memories survived in better shape than did those of animals eating a "normal," non-enriched diet.[119]

That's a slap in the face to conventional doctors who say supplements are a waste of money – just a way of creating "expensive urine" – ha ha. If you listen to them you will pay a dreadful price and forgo many added years of good, healthy life.

According to Alex Richardson, Ph.D., senior research fellow at the Centre for Evidence-Based Intervention at the University of Oxford in the UK, all of us should be taking fish oil supplements and consuming wild (not farmed) fish. Farmed fish are lower in DHA and EPA. Wild fish, of course, raise the issue of mercury contamination, so it's safer to rely on supplements that promise they're free of heavy metals.

Richardson points out that the average American daily consumes only 1.6 grams of omega-3 fatty acids, of which only two-tenths of a gram are DHA or EPA.

To protect your cardiovascular system, the American Heart Association recommends a half gram (500 milligrams) of DHA and EPA each day for healthy adults and .9 grams a day for people with heart disease. That translates to one fatty fish meal per day, or one daily fish oil supplement.

Eating fish every day would be heavy going for most people, and mercury contamination is a concern, so supplements sound like a better choice.

Dr. Richardson recommends 500 milligrams of omega-3 fatty acids a day for children and one gram a day for pregnant women to ensure that youngsters' brains develop correctly.[120]

---

119 https://www.ncbi.nlm.nih.gov/pubmed/24445040
120 http://www.ift.org/newsroom/news-releases/2013/july/16/nutrition-gap-in-omega-3-fatty-acids.aspx

Gallic Acid

Gallic acid is a natural chemical found in a wide variety of food and drinks that's powerfully good for your body and brain. It has **antioxidant** properties that bolster your body's defenses against daily damage caused by everyday toxins and free radicals…

Its **anti-inflammatory** properties defend your cells and neurons from the damage caused by oxidation, and it has **antimutagenic** properties that work to prevent DNA mutations that are often caused by exposure to things like toxic chemicals, too much radiation and ingesting heavy metals like arsenic and cadmium.

Research indicates this hard-working phytochemical can protect your brain from developing dementia – and other health problems, too.

Helps protect against stroke damage

Ischemic injury is damage to the brain caused by blockage or a clot in the blood vessel that can lead to a stroke. **Reperfusion injury**, also called reoxygenation injury, takes place when the blood supply returns to the tissue after a period of ischemia.

Because the tissue has been starved of oxygen and nutrients during the blockage, when the blood returns it can cause inflammation and oxidative damage, rather than simply helping the tissue return to normal function.

Both of these situations – ischemic stroke and its aftermath – are cause for serious concern.

But a study published in the journal *Brain Research* in 2014 found that gallic acid reduced mitochondrial swelling during reperfusion, which then helped to prevent cell death associated with this damage.[121]

Another study, involving animals, discovered that administration of gallic acid five days before and five days after an ischemic/reperfusion injury reduced the amount of damage to the neurons and had a beneficial effect on stroke-induced disabilities.

The antioxidant effects of the gallic acid helped to significantly reduce harmful outcomes like damaged ability to walk, sensorimotor disorders and hypoalgesia (a dulled sensitivity to pain).[122]

Gallic acid for dementia prevention

Scientists have conducted several studies on gallic acid's effect on the hippocampus in relation to Alzheimer's disease.

---

121 https://www.ncbi.nlm.nih.gov/pubmed/25251593
122 https://www.ncbi.nlm.nih.gov/pmc/articles/PMC4075730/

A 2013 study published in the journal *Bioorganic & Medicinal Chemistry Letters* found that gallic acid was the most active compound to inhibit amyloid fibril formation and prevent the clumping and aggregation that follows, which contributes to neuron death.[123]

Other studies back this up. A study of Alzheimer's in mice, published in the April 2016 issue of *Basic and Clinical Neuroscience*, researched the effects of gallic acid on the hippocampus after it's been damaged by beta-amyloid plaques.

The study found that mice treated with gallic acid had better cognitive functioning and less neuronal damage than those that went untreated. Researchers concluded the free-radical scavenging properties and ability to decrease formation of beta-amyloid plaques was responsible for the beneficial effects of gallic acid.[124]

Delicious ways to get more gallic acid

Gallic acid is abundant in many fruits and herbs. Some of the highest levels of gallic acid are found in:

- Strawberries
- Mangoes
- Figs
- Grapes
- Bananas
- Tea, especially black tea
- Cloves
- Wine vinegars
- Apple cider vinegar

When choosing vinegars, go for apple cider vinegar with the "mother" – vinegar starter that contains live, fermenting bacteria cultures[125] – and slow-aged red wine vinegars.

According to a study published in the August 2008 issue of *Food Chemistry*, **red wine vinegar aged in chestnut wood barrels** had the highest concentrations of gallic acid, followed by those that were aged in oak and cherry wood barrels. The phenolic compounds in the wood help to increase the gallic acid already present in the grapes.[126]

And, of course, always choose organic fruits and teas whenever possible.

---

123 http://www.sciencedirect.com/science/article/pii/S0960894X13011451
124 https://www.ncbi.nlm.nih.gov/pmc/articles/PMC4892325/
125 https://www.ncbi.nlm.nih.gov/pubmed/25648676
126 https://www.researchgate.net/publication/222683970_The_phenolic_composition_of_red_wine_vinegar_produced_in_barrels_made_from_different_woods

Garlic

The vegetables in the genus *Allium* are full of medicinal properties and have been used as such for thousands of years. This group of foods includes leeks, onions, scallions, shallots, and chives.

While all members of the genus have benefits, **garlic** stands out from all the others. It qualifies for that overused term "super food" because it's packed with such potent antibacterial, antioxidant and anti-inflammatory properties…

And there's plenty of specific proof that it's good for brain health and cognition.

This amazing, fragrant vegetable can protect your brain and memory from the ravages of dementia.

I just called it fragrant but some may prefer to call it smelly.

Whatever your opinion, its benefits are powerful. According to some sources, Hippocrates, the "father of medicine" himself, recommended garlic for treating respiratory problems, parasites, poor digestion and fatigue.

Garlic can help blood flow to the brain

Garlic is rich in an organosulfer compound called **allicin**, which is part of what gives garlic its power. Allicin is also responsible for garlic's pungent odor when crushed or chewed.

The good news is that if you don't like the taste of garlic or have a problem digesting it, a study published in *The Journal of Nutrition* finds than an **antioxidant-rich aged garlic extract (AGE) can provide many of the same benefits**.

According to the study, AGE is a standardized and highly bioavailable supplement produced by extracting and aging organic garlic at room temperature. The process converts the "difficult" aspects of allicin into something more palatable, while keeping a high level of antioxidants and organosulfer compounds.

The same study found that AGE increased microcirculation, which helped blood flow more freely. This means **garlic can reduce the risk of vascular dementia**, a non-Alzheimer's type of dementia that happens when neurons die because of insufficient blood flow to the brain.

Reduce your risk of heart disease and Alzheimer's disease at the same time

The compounds in garlic have been proven to reduce risk factors for heart disease, many of which also contribute to Alzheimer's disease and dementia. Garlic has been shown to:

- Lower cholesterol (high cholesterol is associated with elevated beta-amyloid plaques)
- Lower homocysteine levels
- Reduce blood pressure and hypertension
- Soothe chronic inflammation
- Destroy free radicals to reduce oxidative damage

Garlic can prevent cognitive decline

In addition to those benefits, AGE shows brain-specific benefits such as protecting neurons from apoptosis (natural cell death) and beta-amyloid neurotoxicity, which **"may help prevent cognitive decline… and improve learning and memory retention."**[127]

A study published in *Current Medicinal Chemistry* found that **S-allyl-L-cysteine (SAC), an active compound in AGE, can prevent the neuroinflammation that leads to the death of synapses.**[128] Keeping synapses healthy is essential to preventing memory loss and cognitive decline.

An in vitro study published in *Phytotherapy Research* found that a **raw garlic extract could inhibit the formation of beta-amyloid plaques**, prompting researchers to conclude that "consumption of garlic may lead to inhibition of beta-amyloid aggregation in the human brain."[129]

A mouse study performed in Tokyo on the effects of AGE found the ones that received garlic had brains that aged slower than the control group.

AGE-fed mice had more brain matter overall, showed better memory and learning, and had less atrophy in the frontal lobe. Maintaining frontal lobe integrity can help **reduce the risk of developing frontotemporal dementia**.

The researchers concluded that AGE "prevents physiological aging and may be beneficial for age-related cognitive disorders in humans."[130]

Garlic stops overactive brain "janitors"

There's yet another chemical in garlic, besides allicin and SAC. It's a carbohydrate derivative known as FruArg. Studies show FruArg can stop overactive microglia cells brought on by chronic inflammation.

---

127 Garlic reduces dementia and heart-disease risk.
128 The "Aged Garlic Extract" (AGE) and one of its active ingredients S-Allyl-LCysteine (SAC) as potential preventive and therapeutic agents for Alzheimer's Disease (AD).
129 Garlic extract exhibits antiamyloidogenic activity on amyloid-beta fibrillogenesis: relevance to Alzheimer's disease.
130 Anti-aging effect of aged garlic extract in the inbred brain atrophy mouse model.

Microglial cells are the "janitors" of the central nervous system. Under normal conditions, they come in and "sweep away" damaged or dying neurons and other cells, leaving room for new cells to grow.

But chronic inflammation causes the microglia to become too active, which produces too much nitric oxide. This in turn causes neuronal damage, setting the victim up for neurodegeneration, Parkinson's disease, Alzheimer's and dementia.

However, a study performed at the University of Missouri School of Medicine in Columbia, Missouri found that **FruArg from garlic extract soothed neuroinflammation and reduced nitric oxide production**. The nutrient works by regulating the expression of proteins in the brain associated with oxidative stress.[131]

How to reap the benefits of garlic

If you already enjoy eating garlic, don't stop! When cooking with it, you'll retain more nutrients by adding it at the end of the dish. High heat breaks down the beneficial compounds.

Crushed raw garlic is great in uncooked dishes like homemade pesto sauce, hummus and salad dressings. You'll get the brain- and heart-healthy compounds and flavor without the overpowering experience of eating a raw garlic clove. Important: it's necessary to crush or chew the garlic to release allicin. Whole garlic cloves will give you less of this precious nutrient.

If you dislike the taste or smell of garlic, or if it upsets your stomach, the AGE supplement is a great way to get the benefits without the smelly "side effects."

Gastrodin

The root of an exotic orchid has been used for thousands of years in China to relieve pain, control convulsions and treat vertigo. Now, in modern scientific studies, it has demonstrated remarkable cognitive benefits. In fact, it looks like a wonder herb.

Whether it's to improve blood flow to the brain, defend against toxicity, preserve memory or promote self-healing, this flowering plant seems to have just about everything you could ask to support brain function.

It's called **gastrodin**.

In lab studies using human and animal cells, researchers from Singapore showed that extracts of gastrodin influenced almost a fifth of the genes that help reorganize and restructure

---

[131] Proteomic analysis of the effects of aged garlic extract and its FruArg component on lipopolysaccharide-induced neuroinflammatory response in microglial cells.

neural connections. This remodeling (plasticity) stimulates processes that give brain cells new life and youth.

When rats were exposed to toxic lead to damage synaptic plasticity in the hippocampus – the part of the brain most associated with memory – the researchers found that gastrodin "can effectively rescue these lead-induced impairments."[132]

Gastrodin has also been shown to influence protein formation and thereby the growth of neurons, as well as a gene that helps brain cells transfer chemical and electrical signals to allow new memories to form.

Protects the brain, reduces inflammation and clears debris

In the lab, gastrodin protected the brain's key learning and memory centers in simulated Alzheimer's and Parkinson's disease. It also increased cell survival and reduced cell death.

A study published in *PLOS One* in 2011 showed that gastrodin can reduce general brain inflammation.[133] The researchers concluded that "gastrodin has a potential as an anti-inflammatory drug candidate in neurodegenerative diseases."

By switching on an enzyme, it can also clear amyloid beta proteins which are associated with Alzheimer's, and even shift biochemistry away from producing them and towards creating normal, healthier proteins.

Boosts blood flow

Rodents that had undergone an ischemic stroke saw blood flow return to normal when gastrodin plus other Chinese medicinal herbs were given 30 minutes after the incident.[134]

In another herbal combination that included gastrodin, 194 out of 202 patients suffering stroke and other brain injuries saw improvement in blood flow.

And 95% of patients with diminished circulation to the back of the brain saw better blood flow when treated with a combination of gastrodin and betahistine (a drug that treats vertigo) compared to 70% in the control group.

Rebalances neurotransmitters

The brain can become stressed when overstimulated, resulting in an imbalance – too many excitatory neurotransmitters and too few inhibitory ones. Extreme imbalances are seen in neurodegenerative diseases, including Alzheimer's.

---

132 https://www.ncbi.nlm.nih.gov/pubmed/19291610
133 https://www.ncbi.nlm.nih.gov/pubmed/21765922
134 https://www.ncbi.nlm.nih.gov/pubmed/9401957

Gastrodin can raise levels of GABA, the brain's main chemical messenger that calms nerve activity. In one study, gastrodin increased GABA by 34%.

Improves memory

Several rodent studies demonstrated reversal of memory impairments caused by toxic drugs and exposure to aluminum. And another showed improved memory in mice that were supplemented with gastrodin compared to a control group that was not. But the most impressive demonstrations were seen in human studies.

A common complication of coronary bypass surgery is cognitive decline, thought to be caused by decreased blood flow and oxygen to the brain and increased levels of debris.

In a randomized, double-blind trial, 200 patients received either intravenous gastrodin or saline (a placebo). 42 percent of patients in the control group saw cognitive decline, including substantial memory loss, but only nine percent of those given gastrodin experienced a similar loss. After three months the figures were 31% and 6%.[135]

In a three-month study of patients suffering mild to moderate vascular dementia following a stroke, the 70 patients who received gastrodin granules dissolved in water performed better on tests of mental function and behavior than did the 50 taking a drug used to treat the condition.[136]

There can be few if any natural compounds that demonstrate such a wide-range of neuroprotective properties.[137] It is available as a supplement from a number of companies (Life Extension, for example).

Ginkgo biloba

Merely recognizing the fact that the herb **ginkgo biloba** has been used medicinally for thousands of years in China should give you a pretty good idea of how beneficial it is. Otherwise, why wouldn't its popularity have waned long ago?

Instead, extracts of ginkgo remain hugely popular – especially for memory support. As a matter of fact, ginkgo is one of the best-selling botanicals in both the United States and Europe.[138]

Which is even more impressive considering the fact that the ginkgo tree is considered a living fossil. The ginkgo tree in its present form has been growing on this planet for 270 million years. That makes it the oldest tree in the world. And scientists say it has no other surviving relatives. They're not even sure how it is related to other plants that are growing today.

---

135   https://www.ncbi.nlm.nih.gov/pubmed/21336736
136   https://www.webmd.com/stroke/news/20030611/chinese-herb-may-help-vascular-dementia
137   http://www.lifeextension.com/magazine/2013/ss/broad-spectrum-protection-against-brain-aging/page-01
138   https://www.ncbi.nlm.nih.gov/pubmed/15710790

Impressive medicine

While botanists puzzle over ginkgo's lineage, medical researchers have been busy catching up with what traditional healers have known for ages: Ginkgo can provide impressive help for mind and body.

As a matter of fact, taking ginkgo biloba extract does so many good things that after compiling a joint review study of ginkgo, a team of researchers that combined scientists from both California and China point out that this herbal preparation "could be considered as a multi-target drug."[139]

In the brain, ginkgo can. . .

- Reduce the accumulation of amyloid-B – the problematic protein that builds up during Alzheimer's disease which can interfere with neurons. Ginkgo can also reduce amyloid-B's toxicity.[140]

- Help mitochondria (energy producing units in cells) work more efficiently by acting as a potent antioxidant.

- Improve blood flow to the brain.[141]

- Enhance the transmission and communication of signals among the neurons in the brain.[142]

As for ginkgo's effect on your memory as you age, here, too, studies have found it can have a profound influence on boosting the plasticity of neurons – the ability of brain cells to form new connections and retain new information.[143]

Related to these effects, researchers at the University of Toledo have found evidence that ginkgo can stimulate the production of new neurons – an important factor for enabling aging brains to hold on to memories. And in the brain tissue of folks who have had strokes, ginkgo supports the rebuilding of new neurons after others have been damaged and destroyed.

The Toledo lab test on animals shows that ginkgo increases neurogenesis by accelerating the activity of a gene that helps produce brand new neurons. Changes of this kind in gene expression are termed "epigenetic; epigenetics is a hot new field in medicine and nutrition."

---

139 https://content.iospress.com/download/journal-of-alzheimers-disease/jad140837?id=journal-of-alzheimers-disease%2Fjad140837

140 https://www.ncbi.nlm.nih.gov/pubmed/17167099

141 https://www.researchgate.net/publication/283857212_Dose-dependent_hemorheological_effects_and_microcirculatory_modifications_following_intravenous_administration_of_Ginkgo_biloba_special_extract_EGb_761

142 https://www.ncbi.nlm.nih.gov/pubmed/15212849

143 https://www.ncbi.nlm.nih.gov/pubmed/15212849

Natural chemicals in ginkgo also help neuroprogenitor cells (the stem cells that become neurons) to link up with other neurons and become functional members of neural networks.[144]

With all these brain benefits, it's no wonder that older members of the Chinese royal court were traditionally given ginkgo nuts to chew on to keep their intellectual abilities intact.[145]

Ginkgo for health

Moving on from its brain benefits, other studies reveal further benefits of ginkgo:

Tests show that compounds found in ginkgo leaves may be used against non-small cell lung cancer. The researchers report that it shows the potential to be more effective than some chemo agents.[146]

Research suggests that ginkgo might offer benefits in reducing the risks and effects of age-related macular degeneration, a leading cause of blindness. People in China, Germany, and France already use it for this purpose.[147]

Research in England shows that ginkgo can relieve some of the pain and walking problems caused by intermittent claudication, a painful condition that often results from clogged leg arteries.[148]

Because ginkgo slows blood clotting, it should not be taken if you are on blood thinners like warfarin (Coumadin). It also interacts with ibuprofen. It also should probably not be taken along with aspirin, clopidogrel (Plavix) or heparin – all of which thin the blood. If you regularly take any prescription medications or o-t-c drugs, the safest move is to consult with a knowledgeable practitioner to see if your meds interacts with ginkgo.

Glutathione

Glutathione is your body's master antioxidant. It recycles other antioxidants like vitamin C, enabling them to go back into battle against free radicals. It's vital for a strong immune system and promotes DNA repair. It boosts liver function, plays a major role in detoxifying the body and protects against inflammation.[149]

Mark Hyman, M.D., chair of the Institute for Functional Medicine, describes glutathione as "…one of the single most important chemicals in the human body…critical to recovery

---

144 https://www.ncbi.nlm.nih.gov/pmc/articles/PMC4133771/
145 https://nccih.nih.gov/health/ginkgo/ataglance.htm
146 https://www.ncbi.nlm.nih.gov/pubmed/29190983
147 https://www.ncbi.nlm.nih.gov/pubmed/23440785
148 https://www.ncbi.nlm.nih.gov/pubmed/11014719/
149 http://www.ncbi.nlm.nih.gov/pubmed/11271724

from nearly all chronic illness, to preventing disease and for maintaining optimal health and performance."

It's also of major importance in promoting brain health and preventing Alzheimer's disease.

Although the body manufactures this antioxidant from three non-essential amino acids – glycine, glutamine and cysteine – the population suffers from an "epidemic deficiency" of glutathione. That's because it is depleted by elements that are commonplace in today's world. (A non-essential amino acid is one that the body can make for itself; we don't need to consume it in our food.)

Factors that deplete our supply of glutathione include toxins, stress, a nutritionally poor diet, pollution, medications, infections, radiation exposure and trauma. Glutathione also declines with the aging process.

It's a deficiency that puts us at real risk of chronic diseases including dementia.

But the news gets worse. A gene called GSTM1 is important in producing and recycling glutathione. Yet half the population lacks this gene.[150]

Glutathione heads up the garbage disposal team

Because the brain is highly metabolically active, it produces a lot of waste. Metabolism simply means converting "something" into energy, and there's always a waste residue left over, much the same as a power plant produces energy and waste by burning fuel. Glutathione is in charge of the garbage disposal team.

If there's too little glutathione the refuse won't be collected and cleared away. That spells trouble.

Alzheimer's patients have from 100 to 1000 times more of the toxic protein amyloid beta than they should have. To find out why, researchers studied 12 people with Alzheimer's and compared them to a control group of 12 healthy people. There was no difference in the production of the protein in each group, but those suffering from Alzheimer's had 30% less ability to clear it.[151]

Lead researcher Dr. Randall Bateman said, "I think it tells us that is the major mechanism that is awry in Alzheimer's disease."

In another study the same was found to be true for Parkinson's disease. Lead researcher and cell biologist Ana Maria Cuervo said, "We have found in Parkinson's there are problems in removing abnormal proteins."[152]

---

150 http://www.ncbi.nlm.nih.gov/pubmed/22381228
151 https://www.ncbi.nlm.nih.gov/pubmed/21148344
152 https://www.ncbi.nlm.nih.gov/pubmed/18172548

Glutathione is your most important antioxidant

Another important mechanism in the development of Alzheimer's comes from the harm caused by free radicals.

Many laboratory and human studies confirm this, and also demonstrate reduced activities and levels of antioxidants in the brains of people with mild cognitive impairment (MCI) as well as Alzheimer's.

A recent review in the *Journal of Alzheimer's Disease*, entitled "The Emerging Role of Glutathione in Alzheimer's Disease," said that "Alzheimer's Disease-associated alterations in glutathione are not simply indicative of increased free radical-induced stress, but play a causal role in Alzheimer's pathogenesis."[153]

How to build up your levels of glutathione

Although glutathione is produced by the body itself and the body also recycles it, today our bodies are too overburdened to maintain adequate levels without help.

To obtain two of the three building blocks of glutathione – glycine and glutamine – you need adequate amounts of good protein from meats, fish, eggs or dairy products. Raw spinach, cabbage and parsley are good vegetarian sources as well as cauliflower, root vegetables, oranges and wheat flour.

Best sources of cysteine, the third building block, are eggs, onions, garlic, and cruciferous vegetables such as broccoli, Brussels sprouts, cabbage and cauliflower. Nuts and seeds are also good sources.

A number of metabolic processes in the body need to be fully functioning to make sure you produce and maintain good levels of glutathione. For most of these processes certain nutrients are required.

You need B vitamins, particularly B2, B6, B12 and folate, as well as zinc and selenium.

To help the body recycle glutathione you need anthocyanins from berries, resveratrol from red wine and alpha lipoic acid from red meat, organ meat, spinach and broccoli.

Why not just take glutathione as a supplement? Unfortunately it is poorly absorbed. Even when given intravenously it's degraded before it reaches the cells. The supplement N acetyl cysteine (NAC) increases glutathione levels and has become popular for this reason.

A proven way to dramatically increase cell levels is to take bioactive, un-denatured whey protein. This has the added benefit of containing ten immunoglobulins that support brain immunity.

---

[153] http://www.ncbi.nlm.nih.gov/pubmed/24496077

Whatever way you choose to maintain high levels of glutathione, you can be sure you are giving yourself powerful protection against the onset of dementia as well as many other degenerative diseases.

Gotu kola

There's a marked difference between traditional medical herbs from cultures around the world and the prescription medicines developed by conventional medicine. **Gotu kola** is a plant remedy that's a case in point.

It's an Asian botanical that's used to protect the nerves and the brain. Some researchers believe it may be helpful in fighting Alzheimer's disease and Parkinson's disease.

Gotu kola's benefits for improving memory as well as for helping to heal skin wounds have been recognized by the Commission E of the German Ministry of Health, the World Health Organization and the European Pharmacopeia.

While modern pharmaceutical companies search for single, powerful compounds that might rescue aging brains from a faulty memory, this medicinal plant contains *thousands* of different substances that affect the body synergistically. According to reports, it produces holistic, wide-ranging effects in physiology.

The herb gotu kola is not related to caffeine-containing cola drinks, nor is it linked to the kola nut. It's an herb that has long been utilized in Ayurvedic medicine, the traditional medical practice in India, as well as in traditional Chinese medicine.

Traditional medicine attributes a dazzling array of benefits to gotu kola – and modern science has begun to study them during the past 20 years. Possible effects include antioxidant support, anti-inflammatory action, immunostimulation, cardiovascular protection, sedation, liver protection, antibacterial defense, anti-fungal activity, relief for varicose veins, and anti-tumor activity.

As researchers have noted, gotu kola "contain(s) a vast number of compounds belonging to different chemical classes." But research so far has focused on the predominant compounds that belong to a class of chemicals known as triterpene saponosides.

Help for aging brains

Gotu kola's protection of an aging brain has been primarily linked to two of the triterpenes generally known as asiatic and madecassic acids.

In lab tests, these substances were shown to inhibit enzymes that break down the neurotransmitter acetylcholine.[154] Because a drop off of the brain's supply of acetylcholine is a symptom of Alzheimer's disease, protecting this neurotransmitter from destruction by enzymes is believed to help the brain hang on to its intellectual capabilities.[155]

Similar lab findings have provided encouraging news for gotu kola's action against Parkinson's disease. Tests show that the herb's compounds can inhibit an enzyme called tyrosinase. Left unchecked, an excess of tyrosinase may break down material in the brain that's needed to keep neurons functioning properly.

Although there haven't been many clinical tests of gotu kola on humans, a few have been conducted that show promise. In a study of about 60 senior citizens, average age 65, who had memory problems (mild cognitive deficiency), a gotu kola extract of 500 mg taken twice a day for six months produced significant improvement in mental capacity.[156]

Heed these warnings!

Although globally gotu kola is one of the best-selling herbs, it can have problematic side effects. Used on the skin it can cause rashes. If you are a man or woman of childbearing age, it can interfere with fertility. It should not be used by pregnant women because it may lead to spontaneous abortion. It should also not be consumed by women who are breastfeeding.

If you have diabetes, metabolic syndrome or very high triglycerides (blood fats), you should consult your healthcare provider if you decide to try gotu kola. It may increase your blood sugar and blood lipids (fats).

Experts recommend not taking gotu kola for more than six weeks at a time without taking a two-week break. We haven't interviewed any doctors who employ this herb in their practice, so please consider this article information, not a recommendation.

But if further studies validate the claims, this intriguing herb offers remarkable benefits. And keep in mind, in Sri Lanka, elephants are believed to live to a ripe old age because they consume gotu kola.

And maybe that's also why – as the saying goes – they never forget.

---

154 http://www.ncbi.nlm.nih.gov/pmc/articles/PMC3359802/

155 Orhan G, Orhan I, Şener B. Recent developments in natural and synthetic drug research for Alzheimer's Disease. Letters in Drug Design and Discovery. 2006;3(4):268–274

156 Tiwari S, Singh S, Patwardhan K, Gehlot S, Gambhir IS. Effect of Centella asiatica on mild cognitive impairment (MCI) and other common age related clinical problems. Digest Journal of Nanomaterials and Biostructures. 2008;3:215–220.

Grape Seed Extract

Natural compounds found in grapes and grape seed extract are proving their mettle in a growing body of research into how Alzheimer's begins and how it might be prevented. And it's interesting that different parts of grapes have different types of benefits.

One of the natural chemicals in grapes thought to be most beneficial for the brain is a group of substances known as polyphenols. Lab tests show they can slow down the destructive processes that damage the brain and bring on dementia.

Stop the first stages of brain loss

One of the initial steps in the breakdown of brain connections that leads to Alzheimer's entails the misfolding of a protein in the brain called tau. For reasons that scientists haven't been able to explain yet, this abnormal formation of tau spreads in the brain, accumulating in one brain cell after another.

When researchers at the Mount Sinai School of Medicine performed lab research on the mechanisms behind this brain tissue damage, they found that misfolded tau is released by brain neurons and then spreads by being absorbed by surrounding brain cells. As it's absorbed, it corrupts other protein that was behaving normally before coming into contact with this destructive substance.

When the scientists treated brain cells in the lab with polyphenols extracted from grape seeds, they found that these natural chemicals could halt this disruptive process.[157]

While some people may swallow the seeds when they eat grapes, supplements are an easier way to get a clinical dose of grape seed extract. Grape seed extract has also been shown to have a powerful effect against cancer. In fact, this unlikely-sounding nutrient may be one of the most exciting discoveries in years.

"Pathology in neurodegenerative disorders is thought to be initiated decades before disease onset," says researcher Giulio Maria Pasinetti. "While further research is needed in humans, we hypothesize that this grape-derived compound may be a promising therapy for not only treating but preventing neurodegenerative disorders involving tau neuropathology."

Keep in mind that results in lab-grown brain cells are not the last word. Human studies are needed to confirm the benefits.

---

[157] http://www.ncbi.nlm.nih.gov/pubmed/21196065

Don't Worry, the Juice Helps Your Mind, Too

Research by Robert Krikorian at the University of Cincinnati College of Medicine has demonstrated that drinking grape juice may also supply enough of these types of polyphenols to help boost memory and language skills in senior citizens whose intellectual abilities have started to slip.[158]

In one test, older adults suffering mild cognitive impairment (MCI) were given grape juice to drink every day for about three months. When they were tested afterwards, their verbal memory had improved and scans of their brains also revealed what appeared to be improved brain function. Spatial memory was also boosted.

Consequently, Krikorian recommends that anyone who wants to protect brain function should include grapes and grape juice in the daily diet. At the same time, he says he would "recommend first of all thinking about eliminating the negative things. I would recommend eliminating as much as possible, and entirely if the person can do it, if they have enough willpower and conscientiousness, to eliminate all processed carbohydrates. So in terms of carbohydrate consumption eating only fruits and vegetables and not consuming grain products of any sort and certainly not sweets of any sort."[159]

In Krikorian's view, foods made from grains, even those made with whole grains, contain overly concentrated amounts of carbohydrates without providing the kind of protective nutrients found in grapes.

The type of research Krikorian has performed supports the idea that an anti-Alzheimer's program can benefit from including grapes and grape seed extract. As Krikorian notes: "They have antioxidant effects… they improve the resilience of neurons, brain cells, to certain kinds of insults like radiation and toxins. They have been shown to actually modify, in a beneficial way, signaling between nerve cells, specifically in memory centers in the brain."

Green Tea

Green tea is a powerful antioxidant widely known for its range of health benefits, including its ability to fight cancer and reduce systemic inflammation. It's a beverage humans have been enjoying for nearly 5000 years. In fact, its popularity in Asia makes it the most-consumed drink in the world.

---

158 http://www.ncbi.nlm.nih.gov/pubmed/20028599

159 http://www.prescription2000.com/Interview-Transcripts/2010-02-12-robert-krikorian-phd-memory-grapejuice-transcriptpdf.html (Reference accessed at time of original publication; may no longer be available.)

And now we know its inflammation-fighting power extends to the brain. As I'll show you in a minute, regular green tea drinkers have *half the rate of Alzheimer's disease* that non-drinkers do.

What's the secret that explains green tea's amazing range of health benefits? Scientists attribute them to a high concentration of micronutrients called polyphenols.

Catechins, a sub-group of polyphenols, are powerful antioxidants proven to scavenge free radicals and fight inflammation. (You know that a tea is high in catechins if it has an "astringent" mouthfeel.)

One particular catechin called epigallocatechin-3 gallate (**EGCG**) makes up about half the polyphenols of green tea. It's piqued the interest of scientists over the past few years ... especially for its potential as a neurotherapy i.e. a brain medicine.

As always, the first question to ask about a potential natural brain-booster is whether the active ingredient is able to cross the VIPs-only, "velvet rope" called the blood-brain barrier.

The news is good: There is no doubt that the blood-brain barrier recognizes EGCG as a VIP. A 1998 Japanese animal study published in the journal *Carcinogenesis* showed EGCG is present throughout the body, including the brain, within one hour after it's ingested ... and considerable amounts remain in the body up to 24 hours later.[160]

This implies that if you drink green tea regularly or take a green tea supplement you maintain effective levels of EGCG in the brain.

But EGCG is more than just a potent anti-inflammatory. It takes brain health to a whole new level.

Alzheimer's prevention, treatment, and recovery

As you know, both neuroinflammation and sticky amyloid beta plaques in the brain are implicated in Alzheimer's disease. They cause neuronal death and loss of brain tissue.

There is convincing evidence that EGCG has the ability to not only reduce inflammation, but prevent and even help brain tissue recover from amyloid plaques if you already have them:

It effectively prevents development of amyloid plaques from two angles. A 2005 study showed EGCG blocks precursor proteins the amyloid proteins require to form ... and a 2006 study confirmed it inhibits amyloid fibrils (base units of the plaque) from forming.[161, 162]

It prevents proteins that have formed from aggregating into the dangerous, sticky plaques.[163]

---

160 http://www.ncbi.nlm.nih.gov/pubmed/9806157
161 http://www.ncbi.nlm.nih.gov/pubmed/16177050
162 http://www.ncbi.nlm.nih.gov/pubmed/16420415
163 http://www.ncbi.nlm.nih.gov/pubmed/23426629

And EGCG has been shown to promote neurogenesis, or the formation of new neurons, by supporting the brain's neuron-creating stem cells ... especially when combined with carnosine, blueberries, and vitamin D3.[164]

It appears that green tea has the power to fight Alzheimer's from every angle, making it a valuable addition to your daily brain-boosting routine.

Quality always counts

As you can probably guess, drinking a cup of green tea is different than taking a concentrated extract in a supplement.

For example, a dried green tea leaf is between 20% and 45% polyphenols by dry weight. But when steeped in hot water, only 5% of those antioxidants actually end up in your teacup. So you ingest approximately three mg of EGCG per cup of tea. It sounds small, but remember the polyphenols work in your body up to 24 hours.

By the way, I'd avoid bottled teas you find in convenience stores if you're after health benefits. According to research presented at the 2010 American Chemical Society conference, some bottled teas have less than 5% of the polyphenol content of a single cup you'd brew at home ... plus, they often contain sugar, artificial sweeteners, colors, or other additives.

These additives may be causing more inflammation and harm than the benefits of the tea can mitigate. But as long as they're not sweetened, they make a much better grab-and-go beverage than soda or a sports drink![165]

A somewhat dubious study of green tea's benefits

There's no doubt that green tea is a powerful, multifaceted anti-aging remedy. However, it's important not to get ahead of ourselves or attribute "magical" results where there's no proof.

I'm thinking of a very small, recently published Swiss study on green tea extract that got a lot of attention from the media because it had a novel twist. The researchers observed human subjects while they were undergoing functional MRI (an MRI that can read brain scans while tasks are being performed.)

The researchers hypothesized that green tea extract increased cognitive function, specifically *working memory*, what we call "short-term memory," where new information is processed and stored.

Once a week for four weeks, 12 men were given 13.75 g or 27.5 g of green tea extract (or none as the control group) via feeding tube. Memory tests were given while the men were examined by functional MRI.

---

164 http://www.ncbi.nlm.nih.gov/pubmed/18260778

165 http://www.acs.org/content/acs/en/pressroom/newsreleases/2010/august/bottled-tea-beverages-may-contain-fewer-polyphenols-than-brewed-tea.html

A sudden surge in brain power – but maybe for the wrong reason

The results led the researchers to believe the green tea extract was increasing the "brain's effective connectivity," that is, the influence one area of the brain exerts over another. This increased "whole brain" connectivity resulted in better performance on the working memory tests.

There are several problems with this study, but the main one is the researchers did not use pure green tea extract. The "test fluids" contained milk whey, other vitamins and minerals, and both sugar and artificial sweetener.

And beyond that? They didn't decaffeinate the green tea extract! At 5% to 10% caffeine, that means participants were given between 68 mg and 275 mg of caffeine – the equivalent of one to four cups of coffee, delivered straight to the stomach. That would be quite a shot to anyone's cognition!

I have a strong suspicion the increase in cognitive function was from the caffeine, not the EGCG. Confirmation would require a larger study using decaffeinated and pure extracts at levels normal people would be taking (about 3 mg EGCG per cup of green tea). The authors wisely noted this issue at the end of their paper.

Bottom line: It's important to check your facts – and also to use your own good sense.

The enzyme factor

Green tea also has an important benefit in the way it affects enzymes that may be related to the development of Alzheimer's disease.

Two enzymes called AchE and BchE break down acetylcholine, an essential neurotransmitter that communicates information between nerve cells in the brain. As we age, we produce less acetylcholine, and with this decline, our memories start to fade.

Drugs that could block these enzymes would be a significant boost to preserving memories. In fact, the best-selling (and largely ineffective) Alzheimer's drugs Aricept and Namenda are AchE inhibitors.

But a study published earlier this year showed there's no need to develop drugs (unless your motive is to make bundles of money). Green tea can produce a similar effect.

In the study, the researchers found that polyphenols in green tea bind with both AchE and BchE. This stopped the enzymes breaking down acetylcholine, thereby increasing levels of the neurotransmitter.

And this is just one way green tea benefits cognition. There are many others. In recent years scientists have found EGCG, the most abundant polyphenol in green tea and also the most potent, works to protect neurons in nine different ways.

Besides preserving acetylcholine, it can also prevent the formation of dangerous amyloid plaques that damage and kill brain cells – as I mentioned above. It can also break down existing plaques and trigger the production of new neurons in the hippocampus, a key area for memory.

That's a lot of brain-healthy support for one drink.

Green tea reduces risk of cognitive decline by more than half

Thousands of lab studies are all very well, but what we really need to know is whether green tea is effective in people.

As recently as 2006 there was no human data available, so Japanese researchers looked at the association between green tea consumption and cognitive function in 1003 people aged 70 or over.

They found that those who drank two or more cups of green tea per day reduced their risk of cognitive decline by 54% as compared with a reduction of only 13% for those drinking black or oolong tea. Those in the study who only drank coffee saw their cognition decline slightly. (I doubt if the finding about coffee will hold up in further study.)

In 2011 scientists tested green tea extract together with l-threonine, another component of green tea, on 91 people with mild cognitive impairment or MCI, a condition that's often a precursor to Alzheimer's disease. The extract was found to significantly improve memory and attention compared to the placebo group.

While these studies are interesting, they don't provide solid evidence for effectiveness, so scientists went one step further by using neuroimaging scans.

Watching the brain in real time

Volunteers consumed a drink containing either green tea extract or placebo. They then had their brains scanned using functional magnetic resonance imaging while completing tasks designed to stimulate memory.

Scientists witnessed a significant boost in activity in the dorsolateral prefrontal cortex in the green tea group. This is the area of the brain needed for processing working memory. It facilitates tasks such as reasoning, learning and understanding language.

A follow-up study by the same research group found green tea extract enhanced frontoparietal connectivity during a working memory task.

The frontoparietal system communicates with many systems throughout the brain and is involved with highly adaptive control processes. It's thought to play a critical role in promoting and maintaining mental health.

There's every reason to believe – based on a solid base of lab research, as well as from watching its real time effects on the brain – that green tea is the real deal, with one word of caution.

While studies usually use extracts of green tea, these may not be as safe as drinking it. Within herbal supplements, the extract has been implicated in many cases of liver injury although no direct association has been found. Our sister company, Green Valley Natural Solutions, decided not to offer green tea extract capsules after looking at the research indicating toxicity.

Until we learn more, it's best to get all the benefits of green tea from the drink itself.

Health idea: Switch from soft drinks to green tea

I prefer coffee and black tea, so for me it's a tall order to give those up and switch to the large amounts of green tea you need to get a therapeutic effect.

But if you're in the habit of drinking soft drinks, you may have an advantage: just substitute green tea instead. In contrast to green tea, soft drinks can do awful things to the body and to brain cells.

One of the main problems with soft drinks is the high-fructose corn syrup that's used as a sweetener. Food manufacturers love to use this syrup because it's so cheap.

But your brain hates it.

Lab research shows, for instance, that getting big doses of high-fructose corn syrup can alter and damage hundreds of genes in the parts of the brain responsible for learning, memory and controlling metabolism (the way the body processes energy).

According to the scientists who have studied this damage, the genetic changes are not only linked to harmful inflammation but can raise your risk for depression, Parkinson's disease and other brain maladies.[166]

In contrast, studies show that green tea can help save the brain from the kind of dysfunction fostered by fructose.

In lab tests, it was shown that while high-fructose corn syrup could harm neurons in the brain, increasing their insulin resistance (keeping them from effectively using blood sugar) and slowing memory, the EGCG from green tea could reverse these effects.

---

166 https://www.ncbi.nlm.nih.gov/pmc/articles/PMC4909610/

Nourishes your neurons

Green tea's ingredients help neurons become less insulin resistant. That's crucial for keeping the brain functioning at full capacity.

A study in Israel, for example, shows that insulin resistance (basically, pre-diabetes) fogs the mind and is linked to a faster decline in memory as you age. That investigation, which tracked the health of about 500 people for twenty years, found that those with the most profound insulin resistance were at the greatest risk of running into significant cognitive complications.[167]

This should not be a surprise. If you've read this far, you know that experts these days say Alzheimer's disease is "Type 3 diabetes". And insulin resistance is the first stage of diabetes. There's more…

- Tests in Japan show that green tea may lower oxidative stress in brain cells, thereby helping them function more effectively.[168]

- Research at the University of Basel in Switzerland shows that green tea improves the connectivity among neurons in the brain and boosts memory.[169]

- A study on the amino acids in tea shows that they can aid in the development of healthier brain function.[170]

- Research at the University of Kentucky indicates that by stimulating the body's increased production of its own antioxidants, green tea can protect brain cells, and other parts of the body, against some of the harmful effects of pollutants.[171]

If mainstream doctors understood its powers, they'd be prescribing green tea for just about everybody.

Cancer prevention

Research at the Arizona Cancer Center shows that the chemicals in green tea can significantly expand production of some of the body's key detoxification enzymes that may affect your chances of developing cancer.

These green tea chemicals, the enzymes known as catechins that I discussed before, increase the production of proteins that are members of the glutathione S-transferase (GST) family. When researchers gave concentrated doses of catechins to about 40 people, they found that it boosted the body's manufacture of these enzymes by up to 80 percent.[172]

---

167 https://www.ncbi.nlm.nih.gov/pubmed/28304291
168 https://www.ncbi.nlm.nih.gov/pubmed/16957869/
169 https://www.ncbi.nlm.nih.gov/pmc/articles/PMC4159594/
170 https://www.ncbi.nlm.nih.gov/pubmed/17904164/
171 https://www.ncbi.nlm.nih.gov/pmc/articles/PMC3946959/
172 http://cebp.aacrjournals.org/content/16/8/1662.long

"(These enzymes) actually convert known carcinogens to non-toxic chemicals, and studies have shown a correlation between deficient expression of these enzymes and increased risk of developing some cancers," says Research Professor H. H. Sherry Chow.

"Expression of this enzyme varies dramatically in people due to genetic variation and environmental factors," Prof. Chow says. "Green tea catechins somehow increase gene expression of these enzymes, which can be an advantage to people with low levels to start with."

Drink green tea, get less cancer

A long list of studies confirms that green tea drinkers generally get less cancer.

When researchers at Chung Shan Medical University in Taiwan analyzed the diets of people with lung cancer and those without, they found that, for smokers, drinking green tea lowered the cancer risk by a factor of more than 12. Overall, among smokers and non-smokers, green tea was shown to lower lung cancer risk by 500 percent.[173]

Scientists at the Vanderbilt-Ingram Cancer Center have shown that green tea lowers women's risk of developing digestive system cancers, especially cancers of the stomach/esophagus and colo-rectum.[174]

"For all digestive system cancers combined, the risk was reduced by 27 percent among women who had been drinking tea regularly for at least 20 years," says Vanderbilt researcher Sarah Nechuta. "For colorectal cancer, risk was reduced by 29 percent among the long-term tea drinkers. These results suggest long-term cumulative exposure may be particularly important."

A tip to make green tea more powerful

To protect your health, the best way to drink green tea is with lemon juice (or take vitamin C at the same time) and just a touch of sugar. Studies at Purdue show that consuming vitamin C (it's in the lemon juice) and sucrose along with green tea can triple your absorption of green tea's helpful catechins.[175]

It's not often that one sees any benefit to eating sugar. In fact, this is the first time I've seen such a benefit reported. I'm a bit skeptical. It's probably the lemon juice-green tea combo that does the trick.

---

173 http://www.aacr.org/home/public–media/aacr-press-releases/press-releases-2008.aspx?d=1730 (Reference accessed at time of original publication; may no longer be available)
174 http://www.ncbi.nlm.nih.gov/pubmed/23053557
175 http://www.ncbi.nlm.nih.gov/pmc/articles/PMC2802066/

Huperzine A

The club moss plant (Huperzia serrata) has been used for centuries in Chinese folk medicine. Now an extract of this plant is showing great promise as a remedy for those who suffer mild to moderate Alzheimer's disease.

It works in a similar way to some of the drugs used to treat Alzheimer's patients, and yet appears to be more effective, safer to use, and its effects last up to twelve times longer. It may also improve learning and memory in healthy people as well, and that's exciting news to those of us who – thank God – don't suffer from dementia and want to keep it that way.

How your brain manufactures a thought

The brain's parietal lobes are its thought factory, responsible for functions such as language comprehension, learning, and immediate memory. And it is in these lobes that acetylcholine, one of the brain's four key biochemicals, is produced. Acetylcholine is required for all the thinking functions I just mentioned, and more.

It's a normal part of aging to see levels of acetylcholine fall, but those with Alzheimer's produce too much of an enzyme called acetylcholinesterase that lowers levels even further, by as much as 90%. A decline that sharp is a disaster. Nerve cells have trouble both sending and receiving signals, leading to serious mental decline.

The main drugs used to treat Alzheimer's focus on blocking this enzyme. Doing so allows acetylcholine levels to rise and cognitive function to improve. And that's what the extract of this ancient Chinese plant called huperzine A is able to do, but much more effectively.

Professor Joel Sussman of the Weizmann Institute in Israel says, "It is as if this natural substance were ingeniously designed to fit into the exact spot in acetylcholinesterase where it will do the most good."[176]

Studies support huperzine A

In one study, about 58% of patients treated with huperzine A showed significant improvement in memory, cognition, and behavioral functions, leading the researchers to say that it "is a promising drug for symptomatic treatment of Alzheimer's disease."

In another study, the researchers concluded that huperzine A is "a safe and effective medicine [that] remarkably improves the cognition, behavior, activities of daily life, and mood of Alzheimer's disease patients."[177]

---

176 http://www.weizmann.ac.il/Structural_Biology/Sussman/
177 http://www.weizmann.ac.il/Structural_Biology/Sussman/

A review of 20 studies[178] published in September, 2013 concluded that "huperzine A appears to have beneficial effects on improvement of cognitive function, daily living activity, and global clinical assessment in participants with Alzheimer's."

Huperzine A has multiple benefits

If being a better enzyme blocker than any prescription drug was the only benefit of huperzine A, it would be impressive enough, but this herbal remedy does even more.

It protects the brain's mitochondria – the energy factories of the cell – from beta amyloid plaques. It is a strong antioxidant, reducing oxidative stress caused by free radicals in the brain. It has the ability to reduce nerve cell death in the brain caused by exposure to a toxin. Huperzine A has even been shown in animal models to promote the growth of nerve cells in the hippocampus, one of the first regions of the brain to suffer damage in Alzheimer's patients.

You don't even need to be middle-aged or elderly to benefit. Huperzine A was also shown to enhance the memory and learning performance of healthy adolescent students.

A comprehensive approach may be needed

Although huperzine A and the other supplements we've talked about are available over the counter, the chemistry of the brain is complicated. A single food or supplement can have a dramatic effect, but each person's needs are unique and it's not totally predictable what individual substance they will respond to.

So don't look at any one nutrient or medicinal substance as a magic bullet that will solve brain health problems all by itself. More often, a comprehensive approach that looks at diet, vitamins, minerals, sleep, exercise and other factors is required to maintain and improve mental health.

That's why this type of medicine is called holistic (or, more accurately) wholistic. By taking a comprehensive approach, many people have reversed mental decline that has already taken place. All that's needed is to put into effect the knowledge we already have about the brain and the natural remedies available, and the results will surely follow, sometimes in a surprisingly short time.

---

178 https://www.ncbi.nlm.nih.gov/pubmed/24086396

Vitamin K

It's been nicknamed "the forgotten vitamin".

Yes, when it comes to vitamins, most of us only know our alphabet from A to E. But there's another one that lies beyond: **Vitamin K.**

Even people who know about this vitamin think we're getting plenty of it in our food, and it only serves one function in the body anyway, so there's no need to consider it further.

Wrong on all counts.

Not only do we need this vitamin for its proven role in blood clotting, but it's now known to be needed for strong bones, flexible arteries and protection against cancer.

And the latest research shows it plays important roles in the brain, too.[179]

As for getting enough K in our food, even this is now questioned. While the average diet may be sufficient when it comes to blood clotting, it doesn't provide enough of this nutrient for the other important functions.

Vitamin K is actually a family of fat soluble nutrients called phylloquinone (K1) and a group of molecules called menaquinones (K2).

K1 is needed for blood clotting and brain health. K2 makes sure calcium is laid in bones and teeth – not in blood vessels where it contributes to plaque build-up in the cardiovascular system and the brain.

Both forms are important when it comes to mental function, but research so far has focused on K1.

Within brain cells K1 is involved with the synthesis of sphingolipids. These are major components of nerve cell membranes and the myelin sheath that surrounds nerve cells. K1 also activates proteins that have important roles in the brain. Insufficient levels of K1 will disrupt wide-ranging functions of the nervous system.

Better cognition, memory and behavior

A study of 320 cognitively healthy men and women aged between 70 and 85 found those with higher blood concentrations of K1 had better brain speed and verbal episodic memory (recall of events that occur within your experience, like where you left your car keys).[180]

---

179 https://www.ncbi.nlm.nih.gov/pubmed/22419547
180 https://www.ncbi.nlm.nih.gov/pubmed/23850343

Of two studies that looked at dietary intake of K1 in seniors, the first found that those with the highest intake scored better on a standard cognitive test and suffered fewer behavioral disorders. The second study found the ones with the highest intake had fewer and less severe subjective memory complaints – i.e. they felt like their memories were working pretty well.[181]

Blood thinners damage the brain

Doctors prescribe anticoagulant drugs – blood thinners – to nearly seven million Americans at risk of heart attack or stroke. Warfarin (brand name Coumadin) is probably the most common. These drugs prevent harmful blood clots. **They work by interfering with the action of vitamin K.**

Does this increase the risk of dementia? Several studies sought to find out.

267 people with an average age of 83 undertook a cognitive test. **Even after taking into account over a dozen factors that could influence the results, the risk of cognitive impairment was 17.4% higher in those who took blood thinning medication.**[182]

Another study of older people taking these drugs found less gray matter volume in the brain including the hippocampus. This means less ability to process information in one of the brain's vital areas for learning and memory and one of the first areas to be affected by Alzheimer's.

In a third study, 7,133 cognitively healthy people aged 65 or above were followed over a period of ten years. Those taking anticoagulants performed significantly worse when it came to visual memory and verbal fluency tests.[183]

Not enough K in our food

1,379 adults living in Ireland were found to have an average daily K intake of 79 micrograms, well below the 120 mcg for men and 90 mcg for women recommended by U.S. authorities as "adequate."

Katarzyna Maresz, PhD., President of The International Science and Health Foundation, writes that "Vitamin K, particularly as vitamin K2, is nearly nonexistent in junk food, with little being consumed even in a healthy Western diet."

John Day is an MD-cardiologist and Medical Director of Heart Rhythm Services in Salt Lake City. He writes that "vitamin K1 and vitamin K2 deficiency is common in the Western world."

---

181 http://www.ncbi.nlm.nih.gov/pubmed/26274973; http://www.ncbi.nlm.nih.gov/pubmed/26923488
182 https://www.ncbi.nlm.nih.gov/pubmed/25151653
183 http://www.ncbi.nlm.nih.gov/pubmed/26576841

It's not hard to get a good intake of vitamin K provided you choose the right foods.

Best sources of K1 are green vegetables such as collards, turnip greens, spinach, kale and broccoli.

If you eat enough K1 to fulfill the body's requirements, it can convert some of it to K2. However, it's better insurance to get K2 from dietary sources. These include fermented foods such as sauerkraut and soybeans, gouda and brie cheese, and grass-fed meat and dairy products.

Lemon Balm

A balm is a preparation that heals or soothes.

And there's an ancient balm with a long history that not only soothes your anxious brain, but may also be able to preserve your ability to think straight and keep your memory working better as you grow older.

Remarkably, this balm – which has been giving people these benefits for thousands of years – has now been shown by medical research to have unique chemical effects on the brain.

The herb I'm talking about is **lemon balm** (Melissa officinalis), a plant that's been used for anxiety and mental support pretty much since people first started using herbs. The plant grows in my garden (in fact, it's pretty invasive – sort of a weed.)

As the name suggests, it tastes and smells just like lemon, and makes a nice addition to tea.

Now we know there's a lot more to it than the flavor. A review of the studies on lemon balm shows it produces measurable benefits for "mood, cognition and memory (that) have been shown in clinical trials."[184]

Valuable for people with Alzheimer's

This venerable herb may be able to help people cope with Alzheimer's disease and slow memory loss.

In a four-month study involving more than three dozen seniors with Alzheimer's disease, investigators tested the effects of taking 60 daily drops of lemon balm extract. The results: folks improved their cognitive abilities on tests of intellectual function while also displaying better mental judgment, longer attention spans, less disorientation, stronger language skills and better reasoning skills.[185]

---

184 http://www.ncbi.nlm.nih.gov/pubmed/27167460
185 http://www.ncbi.nlm.nih.gov/pubmed/12810768

Something new? Not exactly...

For anyone well-acquainted with the history of herbs, this kind of research result shouldn't be a surprise. Way back in the 1500s, a famous physician named Paracelsus was promoting lemon balm as the "elixir of life."[186]

Going back even further to the time of the ancient Greeks, lemon balm was considered essential for dealing with "all complaints supposed to proceed from a disordered nervous system."[187]

Traditionally, the most widespread use of lemon balm has been to treat melancholy (the pre-modern term for depression) and to improve mood. It also has a longstanding reputation as a calming agent that eases anxiety.[188]

These calming effects of lemon balm have now been shown to have scientific validity.

Several studies demonstrate that lemon balm combined with other calming herbs (such as valerian, hops, or chamomile) helps reduce anxiety and promote sleep. A study that examined the herb's effects on people with sleep difficulties discovered that it could help more than four out of five people fall asleep more easily and sleep better.[189]

Another study found that a week of taking lemon balm twice a day caused a significant calming effect, improved mood and greater ability to focus on mental tasks.

Not clear how it works

Exactly how lemon balm produces its benefits in the brain and body is not yet clear. Some of the studies suggest that lemon balm interacts with the important neurotransmitter in the brain known as acetylcholine.

Many researchers believe that when you develop a brain problem like Alzheimer's disease, things go seriously wrong with this neurotransmitter and its receptors in the brain. If lemon balm can help correct this imbalance, that might explain how it tends to get memories and cognitive faculties back on track.[190]

Medical researchers also note that people who develop Alzheimer's are frequently agitated and suffer mood disturbances. Therefore the "specific calming or mildly sedative effect"

---

186 https://theherbalacademy.com/lemon-balm/
187 https://books.google.com/books?id=FDoCAAAAQAAJ&pg=PA222&lpg=PA222&dq=%E2%80%9Call+complaints+supposed+to+proceed+from+a+disordered+state+of+the+nervous+system.%E2%80%9D&source=bl&ots=LPlsZYRoEC&sig=sjTTGgY5iN9wQ0J4LJAuDlXtpp8&hl=en&sa=X&ved=0ahUKEwiS0I7-5pjNAhVGQCYKHY1EA9UQ6AEIHjAA#v=onepage&q=%E2%80%9Call%20complaints%20supposed%20to%20proceed%20from%20a%20disordered%20state%20of%20the%20nervous%20system.%E2%80%9D&f=false
188 https://theherbalacademy.com/lemon-balm/
189 http://umm.edu/health/medical/altmed/herb/lemon-balm
190 http://www.nature.com/npp/journal/v28/n10/full/1300230a.html

of lemon balm could be very useful for folks experiencing these problems.[191]

For my money, the fact that lemon balm can both potentially help the brain stay healthy and relieve the anxiety that is so rampant in today's world makes it a great addition to a supplement regimen. And more than two thousand years of herbalists would agree.

Lemon balm supplements are available on the Internet. Our sister company, Green Valley Natural Solutions, includes a clinical dose of lemon balm in their Vital Force formula, which contains a number of other ingredients and is designed to raise your levels of glutathione (see the article in this book), a vital antioxidant that may be the difference between having a long life or a short one.

Lion's Mane Mushroom

If you're concerned about the health of your brain and avoiding brain-destroying conditions like Alzheimer's disease as you age, be grateful that research into the health benefits of mushrooms has started to pick up speed.

In particular, a peculiar-looking fungus known as lion's mane that grows on downed trees has yielded remarkable compounds that, research suggests, are able to help stimulate neuron development. Studies of lion's mane indicate that its compounds may support the brain's regeneration of the neural connections your brain needs to keep your thinking clear and your memory strong.

Although modern medical studies focusing on lion's mane and other medicinal mushrooms have only been conducted during the past three decades, humans have used lion's mane and other mushrooms for medicinal purposes as well as food for thousands of years.

Ancient Organisms

Mushrooms themselves are one of the oldest types of living things on earth. The wonderful, natural compounds in mushrooms that now generate excitement among scientists are believed to have been more than 500 million years in the making. Mushroom fossils have been discovered in Russia that are thought to be about 545 million years old.

And although most of us picture a mushroom as a lowly fungus sprouting in a cave or on rotting wood, in fact mushrooms that are now extinct once grew up to 30 feet tall.[192]

---

191 http://www.nature.com/npp/journal/v28/n10/full/1300230a.html
192 http://books.google.com/books?id=5nYPdJALMD8C&printsec=frontcover&dq=mushroom+pharmacy&hl=en&sa=X&ei=wkTWUYu4A5Ge9QTzjoHIDQ&ved=0CDMQ6AEwAA#v=onepage&q=mushroom%20pharmacy&f=false

A number of different varieties of mushrooms are known to provide health-boosting natural substances. Of the estimated 1.4 million species of mushrooms that grow on our planet, a mere 80,000 have even been named, much less analyzed for their medicinal value.

Researchers believe that natural compounds found in mushrooms possess the potential to revolutionize our therapies for boosting the immune system and fighting diabetes, heart disease and cancer.

But one of the most exciting areas of research is the way mushrooms support brain health.

In particular, studies of the mushroom called lion's mane (Hericium erinaceus) have uncovered potential for improving the neural networks in the brain. The natural chemicals in this wonderful fungus, according to ongoing research, help the brain regenerate its internal synapse connections. These connections, the internal wiring of the brain, give us our cognitive powers.

When those connections wither and die and are not replaced, the loss is a mental disaster. Those same connections make up the brain cell network that is destroyed by conditions like Alzheimer's disease.

An odd-looking mushroom

As you might expect from its name, the lion's mane mushroom does not look like the toadstools that dot your lawn the day after a summer rain. Instead, this fungus, which generally grows in the hollowed-out sections of fallen trees, produces a mass of white tendrils. To some people they look like a big group of fleshy icicles and to others they look like a big, cartoonish, fungal mop. They have also been compared to an albino lion's mane.

Varieties of lion's mane grow wild in North America. It is popular among mushroom foragers (especially those new to the hobby) because of its distinctive appearance and the fact it grows out of logs. Its habitat and unique look make it unlikely that mushroom hunters will eat a poisonous mushroom by mistake, thinking it's lion's mane. Our research says no other mushroom that grows on wood looks anything like lion's mane.[193]

For medical researchers, the attractive quality of this fungus is its potential strong effect on brains and nerves. It contains previously unknown nutrients that are related to chemicals called nerve growth factors (NGFs).

As the name implies, nerve growth factors help your nerves grow and survive. They also help nerves in the brain and other parts of the body link up and form neural connections. (Until she died at age 103, in 2012, the woman who discovered nerve growth factors, Rita Levi-Montalcini, was the oldest living Nobel Prize laureate. She reportedly used nerve growth factor eye drops daily.)[194]

193 http://themushroomforager.com/2010/09/29/lions-mane-a-foolproof-fungus/
194 http://scientopia.org/blogs/bridgeblog/2012/05/09/a-neuroscience-field-guide-nerve-growth-factor

Incidentally, researchers at Syracuse University report that when you fall in love, your blood levels of NGF increase. According to these scientists, NGF plays a particularly important role in the physiology of the body when you fall in love at "first sight."

The natural substances in lion's mane that stimulate the body's production of nerve growth factors are termed cyathane derivatives. The two types that have been isolated are called hericenones and erinacines.[195]

As mushroom researcher Paul Stamets points out, each variety of lion's mane contains its own unique profile of these natural substances.[196]

NGF deficiency implicated in Alzheimer's

According to experts, a lack of nerve growth factors has been implicated in the development of Alzheimer's disease. When these growth factors sink to low levels, an increasing number of newborn nerve cells in the brain, intended to replace old and decaying cells, die instead at an immature stage of development. As the number of nerve cells dwindles, the brain's networks start to develop holes and gaps.

If this deterioration progresses far enough, your memory also develops gaping holes.

In the view of Japanese researchers who have studied the natural chemicals in lion's mane, the erinacines may be the most potent stimulators of nerve growth factor of any natural compound ever identified.

Researchers look into lion's mane

Although the lion's mane mushroom has been used in Asian medicine for more than a thousand years, it is only during the past two decades that Western medicine has begun to seriously investigate its benefits.

It was in 1991 that Japanese scientists initially discovered that the fungus contained chemicals that stimulate the processes that promote the survival and growth of human nerves.

In 2009, researchers at the Isogo Central and Neurosurgical Hospital in Kanagawa, Japan, gave lion's mane supplements to 30 people who were beginning to have memory problems. After four months of supplements, the mushroom-takers significantly improved their scores on cognitive function tests, demonstrating that their thinking skills had greatly improved.[197]

But after the experiment was stopped, and these people stopped taking lion's mane supplements, their test scores dropped back down to their initial, dismal levels in only a month.

---

195 http://www.mushroomnutrition.com/hericium-erinaceus
196 http://www.huffingtonpost.com/paul-stamets/mushroom-memory_b_1725583.html?
197 http://www.ncbi.nlm.nih.gov/pubmed/18844328

Animal studies point the way

Researchers have given lion's mane supplements to animals whose brains contain the same tangled plaque formations that take shape in the brains of people with Alzheimer's disease. As a result of taking lion's mane, the supplemented animals were better able to navigate mazes compared to animals that had not received lion's mane.

The animals that received the supplement also demonstrated heightened curiosity and an apparent broadened capacity for mental focus and learning about new objects.[198]

Mushroom researcher Paul Stamets terms the reduction in amyloid plaque that occurred when these animals were given lion's mane, to be "remarkable." The amyloid plaques that Stamets commented on are clusters of fragmentary proteins that build up among the dead and dying nerve cells that litter the brain when a person develops Alzheimer's. The presence of these plaques is actually the only known physical confirmation that a patient has Alzheimer's disease (other types of dementia do not necessarily involve plaque formation).

The scientists in Japan said that their lab tests "revealed that H. erinaceus [lion's mane] prevented impairments of spatial short-term and visual recognition memory induced by amyloid β(25-35) peptide."

The brain-boosting molecules in lion's mane

If you want to understand what has researchers so excited about the potential brain-boosting benefits of lion's mane, it helps to understand what mycologists (mushroom experts) study when they tease out fungal natural chemicals.

As I mentioned, lion's mane produces two molecules believed to be nerve growth factor (NGF) enhancers. The factor called Hericenones is produced by the mushroom's fruiting body. The other, termed erinacines, is made in the mycelium.

The fruiting body is the part of the mushroom that yields spores, enabling mushrooms to reproduce. When you see a mushroom sprouting out of the ground, the visible stalk and cap make up the fruiting body.

The mycelium, which takes in food, usually remains underground or, in the case of mushrooms like lion's mane, within a fallen tree. In essence, the mycelium acts like the roots of plants.

Penetrates the blood-brain barrier

One of the most valuable properties of both of the NGF enhancers (Hericenones and erinacines) found in lion's mane is that their molecular properties allow them to cross the blood-

---

198 http://www.imispain.com/blog/wp-content/uploads/2011/12/Mori-K-et-al-2011.pdf

brain barrier. Your body generates its own neuron growth factor itself in the brain (and in other parts of the body), but the chemical structure of NGF renders it too big to enter the brain from the bloodstream.

The purpose of the blood-brain barrier is to restrict the entrance of harmful substances that often include large proteins. Unfortunately, the barrier's protective function often bars access to beneficial substances along with harmful compounds.

But researchers have found that Hericenones and erinacines have low enough molecular weights to allow entry to the brain where they can stimulate the production of neuron growth factor.

Mood improvements

The fact that the nerve growth factor stimulators in lion's mane may improve the structure and function of the brain's neurons is also believed to be the reason studies have shown the mushroom can possibly improve mood and alleviate depression.

When researchers at Kyoto Bunkyo University in Kyoto, Japan, gave lion's mane to more than two dozen menopausal women for a month, they found that it significantly boosted their sense of well-being.[199]

According to the scientists, after taking mushroom supplements the women had fewer menopausal complaints, less anxiety, less depression and were less irritable. They also slept better.

These researchers think that other beneficial chemicals in lion's mane, aside from the nerve growth factor enhancers, were responsible for helping the women who took part in the study.

The scientists conclude that lion's mane "has the possibility to reduce depression and anxiety, and these results suggest a different mechanism from the NGF-enhancing action of [lion's mane]."

Lion's mane roars with brain benefits

The nutrients in lion's mane may be an important tool to stave off the coming epidemic of Alzheimer's disease that threatens the aging population of the United States. The fact that the natural compounds in lion's mane may help the body regenerate neurons and protect the brain's nerve connections as they develop means that the mushroom has the potential to combat a range of neurodegenerative disorders including Alzheimer's and Parkinson's.

Another Japanese study involved seven aging men with dementia who received lion's mane in a daily serving of soup for six months. Six of the seven men experienced notable

---

[199] http://www.ncbi.nlm.nih.gov/pubmed/20834180

functional improvements.[200]

Studies like that one led Paul Stamets to call lion's mane our first "smart" mushroom.

Mushrooms like lion's mane may be the Rodney Dangerfield of nutritious foods: To paraphrase the late comedian, who used to tug at his tie and complain about his lowly status in the world, when it comes to appreciating mushrooms' wonderful health benefits, they don't get no respect, or, at least, not enough. Savvy health consumers know better.

Lithium

Lithium is a neglected supplemental mineral that defends your brain cells as you age. And it's a shame so few people know about it. It can improve your mood, boost personal energy and – perhaps – even offer longer life expectancy.

According to James M. Greenblatt, MD, **lithium** gets just a fraction of the attention it deserves. He calls the mineral a "Cinderella" nutrient because it has been "neglected and ignored."

Shocking as it seems, there's at least one study that shows that lithium, under certain circumstances, might drop your chances of Alzheimer's by a whopping 600%.

That's no typo. A study in Brazil (admittedly, a small study) found that in older people who take antidepressants, taking lithium for that purpose dropped the chances of developing dementia and memory problems by a factor of six.

If you have bipolar depression or similar mood problems, your chances of Alzheimer's and other cognitive difficulties are significantly increased. But it seems that taking lithium – often prescribed for these illnesses – may be able to protect you against this risk.[201]

As I'll show you, there's a ton of evidence that practically every adult should be taking lithium.

Why hasn't lithium won side acceptance as a daily supplement?

It could be because the public thinks of lithium as a drug for schizophrenia and bipolar disorder. It's true that a form of lithium is prescribed by doctors for these ailments. But lithium is not a drug as such, it's one of the basic elements of the periodic table. Healthy people can benefit from it just as we benefit from iron, copper, manganese, chromium and other metals. Lithium is common in the soil and water.

---

200 http://www.fungihealth.com/study-lions-mane-alzheimers-disease
201 http://bjp.rcpsych.org/content/190/4/359.long

As Dr. Anna Fels, a psychiatrist who teaches at Weill Cornell Medical College, notes, "Evidence is slowly accumulating that relatively tiny doses of lithium can have beneficial effects. They appear to decrease suicide rates significantly and may even promote brain health and improve mood."[202]

Traditional healers knew better

Dr. Fels points out that lithium has been used as medicine for hundreds of years (if not longer). For example, Lithia Springs, in Georgia, is the location of natural springs containing high levels of lithium that Native Americans considered a sacred site.

Dr. Fels also mentions that lithium used to be added to beverages. The soft drink 7-Up was originally named Bib-Label Lithiated Lemon-Lime Soda. It included lithium citrate until 1950.

Why did lithium fall out of favor? Blame medical doctors.

After World War II, doctors began dishing out large doses of lithium chloride to patients with heart disease. (They even told them to use this mineral compound as a substitute for table salt.) When people started taking way too much lithium and even doused their steaks with it, many died from the toxic results.

The bad publicity curtailed use of lithium. But the problem was excessively high doses. In small doses, all the evidence suggests lithium is an *extremely* healthy element to ingest.

New research on lithium has started to bring it back into favor

In his book, *Nutritional Lithium: A Cinderella Story*, Dr. Greenblatt explains that the benefits of taking small amounts of lithium as a supplement are varied and without equal. He notes that it's an "essential nutrient for promoting brain health." And it "protects and stimulates the brain in complicated, multi-faceted ways."[203]

Use it to fight inflammation

One of the most important functions enhanced by lithium is protection against inflammation. In fact, lithium is gaining recognition as a joint pain treatment for exactly this reason.

As I've often pointed out, chronic inflammation in any organ leads to serious damage, including damage to brain tissue.

---

202 http://www.nytimes.com/2014/09/14/opinion/sunday/should-we-all-take-a-bit-of-lithium.html
203 Greenblatt, JM & Grossman, K. Nutritional Lithium: A Cinderella Story (2016)

Dr. Greenblatt explains that when inflammation lasts for a short time, it can help heal injured brain tissue by bringing in white blood cells and other healing elements. But uncontrolled inflammation that the body is unable to turn off sets the stage for problems like depression and Alzheimer's disease.

That's why so much medical research is now aimed at figuring out what drives inflammatory processes in the brain's neurons. Controlling these processes can improve brain health and keep neurons from being destroyed by overactive immune cells.

Cytokines are chemical messengers that travel through the body and tell the immune system to increase or decrease inflammation. Lithium can help ease inflammation by slowing the production of the inflammatory cytokines called interleukin-1B and tumor necrosis factor or TNF.

While it curbs cytokines, Dr. Greenblatt explains, lithium can also cut back the destructive actions of microglia, the immune scavenger cells that are supposed to clean up debris from the brain – but which can become over-excited and injure neurons.

For example, research at Boston University shows that during the early development of Alzheimer's disease, microglia can pick up tiny fibers of tau protein – a harmful substance that disrupts the function of neurons in the brain – and release them in a way that causes them to be absorbed by neurons.[204]

But there is some evidence that lithium prevents this destructive process.

This doctor asks, "What are we waiting for?"

Research in Brazil on animals shows that lithium taken during the early development of Alzheimer's may "alter the pathological characteristics" of the disease. So, for Alzheimer's, which conventional medicine can't treat, the researchers believe lithium offers "new hope for the therapeutic treatment of this disease."[205]

Which leads James Phelps, who directs the Mood Disorders Program at Samaritan Mental Health in Corvallis, Oregon to ask, when it comes to using lithium for Alzheimer's prevention – "What are we waiting for?"[206]

May add years to your life

Lab research into lithium's effects on the body also suggest that it may help people live longer.

A study at the University of London demonstrates that low doses of lithium help fruit flies live 16% longer. And the researchers think that lithium can have a similar effect in humans.[207]

---

204 https://www.ncbi.nlm.nih.gov/pubmed/26436904
205 https://www.ncbi.nlm.nih.gov/pmc/articles/PMC4659557/
206 http://www.psychiatrictimes.com/bipolar-disorder/lithium-alzheimer-prevention-what-are-we-waiting
207 https://www.ncbi.nlm.nih.gov/pubmed/27068460

The longevity benefit, they say, is partly related to the fact that lithium blocks the activity of a harmful molecule called GSK-3 (glycogen synthase kinase-3) a substance also thought to be involved in the development of Alzheimer's disease.[208]

But the brain benefits don't stop there: Along with blocking GSK-3, lithium may also play a part in keeping your brain from shrinking.

Jonathan V. Wright, M.D., a pioneer in natural medicine, says in the introduction to Dr. Greenblatt's book that lithium has been shown to help keep your brain larger as you age.[209]

Plus there may even be further benefits to lithium. . .

A Greek study shows that areas with drinking water containing more lithium experience lower suicide rates. The researchers point out that studies show: "… the existence of statistically significant inverse associations between the lithium levels in drinking water and the incidence of suicides, homicides, rapes, possession of narcotic drugs, and in juveniles, the rates of runaway from home."

These scientists urge follow-up research on other studies showing lithium may be useful for Lou Gehrig's disease (the neuro-degenerative illness that inspired the video parade of ice bucket challenges.)[210]

Low doses for healthy people

In the large "pharmaceutical" doses given to bipolar patients, lithium has serious side effects. But in the small doses advocated by Drs. Wright and Greenblatt, problems are rare. I've taken it daily for years.

Lithium orotate, the preferred form, is easily available on the Web, or you can order it from our sister company, Green Valley Natural Solutions – just click here.

Luteolin

Remember the old fable about the boy who cried wolf?

The youngster in the tale gets in trouble for screaming time and time again that there's a dangerous wolf in the neighborhood – when there's no wolf.

His false alarms upset everyone until they learn not to believe him.

---

[208] https://www.ncbi.nlm.nih.gov/pmc/articles/PMC3073119/
[209] https://www.ncbi.nlm.nih.gov/pubmed/21030008
[210] http://www.ncbi.nlm.nih.gov/pubmed/24072668

Well, your brain has a similar warning system – special immune cells called microglia that are supposed to give warning when your brain is threatened by disease-causing microbes.

But just like the boy's false alarms in the old story, things can go wrong with microglia and they can cry wolf when your brain is in no danger. Stick with me on this, because **luteolin**, a nutrient found in celery and other ordinary, everyday foods can stop this harmful process.

In experiments, luteolin nutrient restored the memories of older animals to the same level as younger animals.

When they cry "wolf," the microglia can rush around the brain in a tizzy, trying to fight off a menace that doesn't really exist. The microglia false alarm leads to **inflammation** – i.e. the activation of immune cells that, without microbes to battle, end up injuring brain tissue instead.

There are natural ways, including luteolin, to keep this from happening. Before I get to that, let's take a closer look at what researchers have found out about how overactive microglia can wander into parts of the brain that you need in order to preserve your memories. While mucking about where they're not needed, they short-circuit your intellectual abilities.

Microglia breaking bad

Researchers at Stanford microscopically examined the brains of people who died with Alzheimer's disease. The study discovered that microglia that have scooped up iron can invade the hippocampus, the section of the brain that is supremely important for forming memories.

While the researchers don't know for sure how the iron entered the brain tissue, they think that tiny injuries to the blood vessels that supply the brain may have leaked and allowed it in. The blood's hemoglobin, like all hemoglobin, is rich in iron.

According to the Stanford researchers, these inflammatory microglia are like boys crying wolf, but even worse: imagine the little boys are armed with AK-47s. The trigger-happy microglia are not just shouting about an imaginary foe, they're firing off their immune weapons and destroying brain tissue.

You need to declare a cease-fire

Fortunately, luteolin can persuade these destructive immune cells to calm down and back off.

Researchers at the University of Illinois in Champaign have found that **luteolin**, the compound found in carrots, peppers, celery, olive oil, rosemary, peppermint and chamomile, can persuade your microglia to cool it.

In this research, the scientists discovered that luteolin stops microglia from producing cytokines, immune signaling molecules that set off significant inflammation and cellular damage.

According to researcher Rodney Johnson, Ph.D., "We found previously that during normal aging, microglial cells become dysregulated and begin producing excessive levels of inflammatory cytokines. We think this contributes to cognitive aging and is a predisposing factor for the development of neurodegenerative diseases (like Alzheimer's disease)."

Dr. Johnson's lab tests have revealed that luteolin reins in microglia and prevents the inflammatory processes that kill off neurons.

"The neurons survived (in our tests) because the luteolin inhibited the production of neurotoxic inflammatory mediators," he explains.

And when Dr. Johnson tested luteolin on older lab animals, he found that not only did age-related brain inflammation go into reverse, but he was able to confirm improvement by giving them memory tests. These tests showed their learning abilities got sharper – to the point where they were the equal of younger animals.

That's why Johnson believes that eating a healthy diet filled with fruits and vegetables – and don't forget the celery, carrots and peppers – is key to helping your brain age better.

So the next time you snack, reach for a celery stick instead of a pretzel stick.

Magnesium

How well your brain works depends on how well your synapses work. The synapses are the places where the brain's neurons communicate with each other. As research shows, the reliability and efficiency of these communications depend on abundant levels of **magnesium**.

And it just so happens that about half of us are dangerously low in that mineral. There's good evidence that increased intake of magnesium can improve the function of your synapses and protect your mental abilities against the hazards of aging.

Researchers are becoming convinced that when you run short of magnesium your brain's neurons and cognitive abilities can short out like a malfunctioning electric circuit.

Enhances brain power in young and old alike

A range of experiments during the last few years have shown that magnesium is a brain booster. For example, in tests on laboratory animals, researchers at MIT have demonstrated that magnesium can increase learning abilities and memory.

Using specialized magnesium supplements, Guosong Liu, who is now at the Center for Learning and Memory at Tsinghua University in Beijing, China, has shown that magnesium may enhance brain power in both the young and old.[211]

"We found that elevation of brain magnesium led to significant enhancement of spatial and associative memory in both young and aged (animals)," says researcher Liu.

Liu and his fellow researchers examined how magnesium altered the functional and structural properties of synapses. They found that at any age, magnesium increased the adaptability of synapses while boosting their density in the hippocampus, the vital area that takes part in learning and memory.

"Half the population of the industrialized countries has a magnesium deficit, which increases with aging. If normal or even higher levels of magnesium can be maintained, we may be able to significantly slow age-related loss of cognitive function and perhaps prevent or treat diseases that affect cognitive function," Liu says.

Aided brain development in animal trials

Research at Tel Aviv University in Israel supports the importance of magnesium.[212]

In these tests, scientists compared the cognitive skills of two groups of animals. One was fed a normal diet while the other consumed magnesium supplements with their meals.

Behavioral tests found that cognitive functioning improved in the animals given supplements. These animals also grew extra synapses in their brains. Consequently, their brains were able to more effectively retain memories.

Although the specific supplement used in all of these research projects is not yet available to consumers, the researchers believe that all of us should be making an effort to eat more magnesium-rich foods. The supplements currently on the market are not believed to deliver magnesium very efficiently to the brain.

According to researcher Inna Slutsky of Tel Aviv University, eating meals that contain more magnesium won't help your memory overnight, but if you eat those foods day after day you should experience a gradual improvement. She also believes your magnesium intake can fight the development of dementia and other signs of aging in your brain.

Rich sources of magnesium include dark, leafy vegetables like spinach as well as broccoli, cashews, almonds, and a variety of fruit. If you take in less than 400 milligrams a day, you not only increase your risk of cognitive difficulties, you also increase your danger of heart problems, allergies and asthma.

---

211 https://www.ncbi.nlm.nih.gov/pubmed/20152124
212 https://www.aftau.org/weblog-medicine--health?&storyid4704=1722&ncs4704=3

Melatonin

Taking hormones to fight aging can be an iffy proposition. But there's one anti-aging hormone that is perfectly legal, very safe and that has garnered strong support from cutting-edge medical researchers – **melatonin**. They marvel at its ability to support the aging brain and fight oxidative stress. And this inexpensive hormone is sitting on the shelves of practically every pharmacy in the country.

Now, we're not talking about body builders taking steroids to build muscle, or older women using hormone replacement therapy to stave off the discomforts of menopause. And it's not human growth hormone that many people take to rejuvenate the body.

Supplementing with melatonin, whose production in the body falters as you age, can be a safe way to defend your mental and physical well-being as you grow older.

Taken in appropriate doses, melatonin may help you sleep better and lose weight, effects that are a far cry from the potential cancers, heart problems and disrupted sexual function that may be the unintended results of taking other hormones.

Your body makes this natural substance in the pineal gland, a tiny bean-sized organ within the brain, located in its very center, between the brain's hemispheres.

With the passing years, your pineal gland secretes less and less melatonin. Some researchers believe this falloff in the body's melatonin production is a key factor that makes older people more susceptible to sleep problems and brain dysfunction.

Combine it with this and get even better results

A lab study in Barcelona, Spain, shows that a combination of exercise and melatonin may produce a synergistic benefit that defends the brain against mutations associated with Alzheimer's disease. In this lab test on animals, a melatonin and exercise combination was shown to be effective against the harm linked to three different mutations.[213]

"For years we have known that the combination of different anti-aging therapies such as physical exercise, a Mediterranean diet, and not smoking adds years to one's life," says researcher Coral Sanfeliu. "Now it seems that melatonin, the sleep hormone, also has important anti-aging effects."

The Spanish study demonstrated that melatonin protects brain tissue from oxidative damage and helps defuse impairments linked to amyloid beta peptide, a harmful protein that collects in the brain during the development of Alzheimer's. In addition, the hormone helps maintain the mitochondrial function in brain cells. Mitochondria are the structures responsible for

---

213 http://www.ncbi.nlm.nih.gov/pubmed/22177720

a cell's energy production. Injury to the mitochondria often results in illnesses like Parkinson's disease.

Its important to note that this was an animal study, and human studies are needed to confirm its effectiveness.

"Even though many more studies and clinical tests are still required to assess the doses of melatonin which will be effective for a wide range of diseases, the antioxidant and anti-inflammatory properties of melatonin mean that its use is highly recommended for diseases which feature oxidative stress and inflammation," says researcher Darío Acuña-Castroviejo.

Acuña-Castroviejo believes melatonin can be useful for alleviating epilepsy, chronic fatigue, fibromyalgia, and even the aging process itself.

Best ways to take it

If you decide to take melatonin supplements, experts at the Mayo Clinic caution that it can interact with birth control pills, blood thinning pharmaceuticals, diabetes treatments and immunosuppressants. Those being treated with those types of medications should consult a doctor before taking melatonin pills.

Even more important is the fact that the recommended dose on most melatonin supplements is MUCH too high, and the result can be unpleasant side effects like insomnia, or worse.

Dr. Michael Breus, a recognized expert on sleep and sleep disorders, says, "The correct dose is between a half and one milligram. The 3 mg, 5 mg, 10 mg doses that you see out there in many supplements are all in overdosage format."

It's not easy to find a supplement with a dose as low a one milligram or less, but they do exist. Dr. Breus also advises taking melatonin 90 minutes before you want to fall asleep, because it does not act fast.

In addition, it's not a sedative, it's "a circadian rhythm regulator," and that's a whole different story. Your body produces its own melatonin, and if you don't mess with your natural daily rhythms, your melatonin level is highest at night, falling steadily until the morning, when it's at its lowest point.

Then your levels build up again steadily through the day until bedtime.

This means it's important to know that *light stops the production of melatonin*. So if you have lights in your bedroom, or if you stay up late reading, using electronic devices, watching TV – your melatonin production is thrown off and you likely won't sleep well. Even those little lights on TVs and computers that are ALWAYS on will disrupt your melatonin. You don't want ANY light in the room where you're sleeping.

Melatonin is also found in a variety of vegetarian foods including almonds, mustard, cherries, flax seed, Goji berries, cardamom, sunflower seeds, coriander, fenugreek and fennel.

There's an interesting weight-loss angle to melatonin. Research shows it may encourage the body to make beige fat, a specialized fat tissue under the skin that burns off extra calories. Other studies have shown that melatonin can help reduce triglycerides (blood fats), boost HDL (good cholesterol) and reduce LDL (bad cholesterol).[214]

The ideal is to maintain your natural levels of melatonin with good habits. But a pill can help as long as the dosage is low and it doesn't interact with your medications.

Mushrooms

To the Romans, mushrooms were the "food of the gods." Ancient Greek warriors ingested them before battle to increase their strength. In Chinese culture, they're considered an "elixir of life."

While most people enjoy them as part of their everyday diet, certain varieties of **mushroom** are prescribed in ancient medical traditions for their health and healing properties.

A recent review described mushrooms as exhibiting "antioxidant, anti-tumor, anti-virus, anti-cancer, anti-inflammatory, immuno-modulating, anti-microbial, and anti-diabetic" properties.

That's quite a list of benefits. Let's probe further...

Useful against dementia

The review, which appeared in the *Journal of Medicinal Food* in January, also suggested that mushrooms could play a role in preventing Alzheimer's disease and other age-related neurodegenerative diseases.

The authors, three researchers from the University of Malaysia, summarized the scientific information they were able to find on the brain benefits of eleven different varieties of edible and medicinal mushrooms.[215]

Looking mainly at rodent studies, **they found that each variety boosted the production of nerve growth factor (NGF).**[108]

This protein-like molecule is important for growth, development, survival and maintenance of nerve cells.

---

214 http://canalugr.es/health-science-and-technology/item/49083 : (Reference accessed at time of original publication; may no longer be available.)

215 https://www.gdtimag.com/wp-content/uploads/2017/01/jmf2E20162740.pdf : (Reference accessed at time of original publication; may no longer be available.)

The researchers also found that NGF in turn promoted the regeneration of peripheral nerves - the network that connects the brain and spinal cord.

Because the body uses NGF to build nerve networks throughout the body, this natural body chemical is seen as a key factor in maintaining brain and nervous system health and lowering the risk of cognitive decline.

Some of the most important mushrooms in the review were:

Cordyceps - This has a long tradition in Chinese and Tibetan medicine. It has anti-inflammatory properties and is able to promote neural growth. Other lab studies show the cordyceps mushroom is able to prevent memory loss in rodents and the death of human neurons.

Oyster - The most active compound in this large, edible wild mushroom is uridine, which has been shown to be critically important in many areas of brain function.

Maitake - This species is able to induce neurite outgrowth - the growth of axons and dendrites that project from the body of a nerve cell. Dysfunction of this outgrowth leads to neurodegeneration. Studies have also shown that maitake reduces inflammation, inhibits high blood pressure, and enhances insulin sensitivity.

Reishi - Used medicinally for thousands of years in Asia, this mushroom improves cognitive abilities and could prevent toxicity and death of brain cells. Mice that were fed reishi extract in their food had lower brain amyloid and higher levels of antioxidants.

And reishi can produce some remarkable benefits. It's worth a few additional words...

Known as the "mushroom of immortality," reishi also goes by the name of lingzhi, and its botanical name is *Ganoderma lucidum*.

Polysaccharides and triterpenes are two major physiologically active components of reishi. They have powerful anti-inflammatory and antioxidant properties. Because free radicals and inflammation are hallmarks of diseases like Parkinson's and Alzheimer's, it's logical to infer that reishi would benefit these conditions.

And that's what a number of studies have shown.

In one study reishi mushrooms were demonstrated to reduce the influence of amyloid beta proteins that are the key physical symptom of Alzheimer's. The scientists who conducted the research concluded that reishi "can prevent harmful effects of the exterminating toxin amyloid beta in Alzheimer's disease."[216]

Five studies have shown reishi can protect brain cells from the type of inflammation that causes Parkinson's disease. The mushroom was described as a "promising agent" for the treatment of this condition.

---

[216] https://www.ncbi.nlm.nih.gov/pubmed/18083148

Most of the drugs used to treat Alzheimer's are aimed at blocking acetylcholinesterase. This is an enzyme that breaks down acetylcholine, an essential neurotransmitter. It's believed that high levels of acetylcholinesterase and resulting loss of acetylcholine is an important feature of serious mental decline. The triterpines in reishi have been shown to exhibit "moderate acetylcholinesterase-inhibitory activity."[217]

Reduces stroke damage, protects against diabetes

In the lab, reishi demonstrated that it could benefit the victims of stroke in two ways.

It was able to reduce the stroke-damaged area within the brain, and thus limit the functional and behavioral damage that the stroke caused.

Reishi also protected the brain from attack by free radicals and from injury caused by reduced levels of blood flow and oxygen.

In one study, rats were administered a chemical that's toxic to the hippocampus – an area of the brain that's critical for short and long-term memory. In the three weeks leading up to this trauma their diet was supplemented with reishi. The researchers found the mushroom improved cognitive function, with a significant reversal of the damage caused by the toxin.[218]

The benefits of reishi also extend to diabetes.[219] People with this condition have a much greater risk of not only cognitive decline and loss of brain function, but also cancer and heart disease.

Reishi has been shown to reduce blood sugar levels, improve glucose tolerance and increase insulin sensitivity. In one animal study it was described as "an effective antidiabetic agent." And in a human study it was found to have "mild antidiabetic effects."

Although there is clearly a need for more human studies, reishi seems to be brain protective in a number of critical ways.

But all of the mushrooms I have discussed here "may fulfill a preventive function against the development of Alzheimer's."

According to one member of the team that conducted the mushroom review, Professor Vikineswary Sabaratnam, "Mushrooms contain diverse yet exclusive bioactive compounds that are not found in plants. It's very likely a dietary intake of mushrooms or mushroom-based extracts might improve brain function. Regular consumption of mushrooms may reduce or delay development of age-related neuro-degeneration."

---

217 https://www.ncbi.nlm.nih.gov/pubmed/21924611
218 https://www.ncbi.nlm.nih.gov/pubmed/21242065
219 https://www.ncbi.nlm.nih.gov/pubmed/23874589

NAC (N-Acetyl-L-Cysteine)

Antioxidants play an important role in keeping cells healthy by reducing oxidative stress and its result, inflammation, a major factor in dozens of health problems including cancer, dementia, arthritis and cardiovascular disease.

But so many antioxidants are being touted these days, it can get noisy and confusing if you're not a full-time nutrition expert.

Let me help clear up the confusion a little bit: There's ONE antioxidant – **n-acetyl-L-cysteine** – that will help you for sure.

Just looking at it, **n-acetyl-L-cysteine** sounds like a mouthful. Not to worry: Most people just call it **NAC**.

In chemistry terms, NAC is the "acetylated" (ah-see-tull-ated) form of L-cysteine, an amino acid that contains sulfur.

What you really need to know is that your body can more easily absorb the acetylated form than the pure L-cysteine base. And that's a good thing, because NAC is a powerful antioxidant – a hungry free-radical scavenger – and a detoxifier too boot.

Prevents the death of neurons

One study from the journal *Cerebellum* showed NAC protects against oxidative-stress-induced neuronal death even in granule neurons, tiny cells found throughout the brain.[220]

As you may know, if enough neurons are damaged or killed by oxidative stress, cognitive decline and neurodegenerative diseases like Alzheimer's are just around the corner … which is why getting enough NAC can help on all fronts.

NAC also plays a second important role: helping your body synthesize *glutathione*, another essential antioxidant that fights for healthy, stress-free neurons.[221] Although the body makes its own glutathione, many people – especially older people – are deficient.

It's generally not effective to take glutathione by mouth, because it doesn't survive stomach acid. The strategy nutritionists recommend is to take supplements like NAC that help your body make glutathione. There aren't many such nutrients, and they're priceless for boosting your health and extending your life.

NAC stimulates enzymes within the membranes of neurons that increase glutathione production at the cellular level. This, in turn, restores the neuron's ability to fight damage caused by free radicals – even in smokers who tend to have high levels of inflammation.

---

[220] http://www.ncbi.nlm.nih.gov/pubmed/17853088
[221] http://www.ncbi.nlm.nih.gov/pubmed/17602868

In one study, performed in China, mice were injected with amyloid beta-peptides to produce Alzheimer's disease. (Interestingly, researchers found lower glutathione levels in these mice – another piece of proof that this is a key antioxidant in Alzheimer's prevention.)

After inducing Alzheimer's disease in the mice, the scientists observed them as they ran through different mazes.

Some of the subjects were then given a dose of NAC.

The mice given NAC showed *significantly* greater memory retention and shorter latencies when they went through the mazes again.[222] These findings lead the researchers to conclude that NAC is a potential neuroprotective agent against Alzheimer's disease. Naturally, animal studies are not the last word, and human studies are needed as confirmation. (However, human studies *do* confirm that NAC raises glutathione levels.)

Besides being a powerful antioxidant and precursor to critical glutathione, NAC has been shown to downregulate genes responsible for inflammation … yet another contributing factor to degenerative diseases of the brain and nervous system.

Getting the Right Amount of NAC

Animal protein from pork, chicken, turkey and duck contains cysteine, the precursor amino acid for NAC. Vegetable sources of cysteine include garlic, onions, Brussels sprouts and red peppers. You can also find it in fermented milk products like ricotta cheese, cottage cheese and yogurt.

Unfortunately, NAC itself is not found in food sources, which means a supplement is the way to go.

Most people will benefit from 600 to 1800 mg per day, with recent studies showing it's safe to consume up to 2000 mg per day.

We've seen reports that NAC also prevents cases of avian and seasonal flu, reduces the frequency of COPD attacks, blocks cancer development in nearly every step of the disease, improves insulin sensitivity in metabolic disorder … and more.[223]

It's a great, broad-spectrum antioxidant to have working for you in the long run.

---

222 http://www.ncbi.nlm.nih.gov/pubmed/17602868
223 http://www.lifeextension.com/magazine/2010/5/N-Acetyl-Cysteine/Page-01

Phosphatidylserine (PS)

Phosphatidylserine (PS for short) is a phospholipid – a type of substance in cell membranes that gives cells structure and regulates what can move in and out of a cell. But phosphatidylserine primarily forms a crucial part of the membranes of brain tissue. Myelin – the sheath that covers nerve fibers and influences how fast nerve signals travel around the brain – is particularly rich in PS.

Research on neurons shows that PS plays an important role in supporting memory and brain function. And what's more, studies also indicate that taking PS supplements can help improve intellectual abilities in older people – although sometimes the research also seems to show that the benefits wear off after a while.

In perhaps the most famous PS study, *researchers found a reversal of brain-aging of nearly 14 years* in patients who took the supplement for 12 weeks. The dose was 300 mg per day. The participants improved in learning and remembering written information, remembering names and recognizing people, and memory of numbers.

Taking 14 years off the age of peoples' brains is enough to get my attention! Apparently many others feel the same way, because PS is one of the most popular brain supplements.[224]

The fact is, your brain can't work very well without PS. And only three parts of the human body produce appreciable amounts of phosphatidylserine –the brain, the kidneys and testis.

Scientists have also learned that PS interacts and links up with docosahexaenoic acid (DHA), one of the omega-3 fats in fish oil, to keep neurons behaving properly. How important is this partnership? Research demonstrates that when someone deteriorates from the pre-Alzheimer's condition called mild cognitive impairment – that is, when memory first starts to slip, but before the person succumbs to full-blown Alzheimer's disease – the amount of DHA and PS in the brain's cerebral cortex also declines drastically.[225] The cerebral cortex is a brain area that controls thoughts and actions.

Apparently, when you're younger, your brain is pretty adept at producing its own PS. But as you get into your 40s and 50s, that capability starts to slip and, instead, the membranes of the brain's neurons begin to incorporate more cholesterol. That substitution may harm brain function and slow your thinking.

---

224 Schreiber S, Kampf-Sherf O, Gorfine M, Kelly D, Oppenheim Y, Lerer B. An open trial of plant-source derived phosphatidylserine for treatment of age-related cognitive decline. Isr J Psychiatry Relat Sci. 2000;37(4):302-7.
225 https://www.ncbi.nlm.nih.gov/pmc/articles/PMC3409580/

The many roles of PS

Among other things, phosphatidylserine is involved in. . .

- The function of dopamine in the brain. Some researchers believe that when phosphatidylserine becomes reduced in the brain, dopamine release is impaired and interferes with memory.

- The production and release of acetylcholine – a neurotransmitter required for memory consolidation.

- The regulation of glucose metabolism for supporting neuron function.

- Controlling stress-related levels of cortisol. A study in Germany shows that taking PS can ease and "normalize" the hormonal reaction to chronic stress.

- The production and release of enzymes that help form memories.[226]

One of the largest studies of PS took place in Italy. About 500 patients who were suffering from moderate to severe loss of memory were given 300 mg of PS daily for six months. The researchers reported that when people were treated with PS they experienced "significant improvements."[227]

And there's evidence that taking PS along with ginkgo can help boost memory and brain function. When researchers in England gave "younger" people (in the write-up of the study they don't say exactly what their ages were) a combination supplement of both phosphatidylcholine and a ginkgo extract, they found that their performance on tests of mental acuity was faster and more accurate. And this was just a one-time dose followed by a written mental test.

The researchers also reported that the herbal combination made their subjects calmer while they were taking the memory tests.[228]

Another combination that may help any older person who is having some memory issues – taking PS along with omega-3 fats from fish oil.

Since, in the brain, PS is combined with omega-3 fats in cell membranes, researchers at the Tel-Aviv Sourasky Medical Center in Israel tried giving a combination of both PS and omega-3 fats to 157 people for 15 weeks. The result? The participants' ability to remember words was "significantly improved." Even the folks in the group whose thinking powers were pretty good when the study started enjoyed improved learning ability.[229]

---

226 https://www.ncbi.nlm.nih.gov/pmc/articles/PMC4220811/
227 https://www.ncbi.nlm.nih.gov/pubmed/8323999/
228 http://www.prohealth.com/library/showarticle.cfm?libid=29840
229 https://www.ncbi.nlm.nih.gov/pubmed/20523044

The common message of all this research is pretty clear: If your memory seems okay but you want to improve, PS can help. And if you're starting to worry about how your brain is working, PS might help you, too. Throw in a little fish oil and ginkgo with your PS and who knows, you might find yourself remembering more than you ever thought you would.

Pomegranate

The pomegranate – as well as pomegranate supplements and/or pomegranate juice – is a botanical marvel every person concerned about brain health should consume. It's a fruit that has long been treasured for it benefits – so valuable in fact, that according to some scholars, the famous forbidden fruit in Genesis was probably the **pomegranate**.

Potent nutrients go to your head

Tests at the University of Rhode Island show the pomegranate contains polyphenols that help defend the brain's neurons against the malfunctions that become more common as you grow older. (Polyphenols are natural antioxidant chemicals that plants use to protect themselves from ultraviolet light and infections, and which the human body uses to boost the immune system.[230])

Although the Rhode Island researchers found that most pomegranate polyphenols couldn't cross the blood-brain barrier, a filtering structure that keeps many substances out of brain tissue, their tests demonstrated that the bacteria in your digestive system can interact with polyphenols to produce **urolithins** – chemicals that *are* able to penetrate the brain.[231]

The lab tests indicated that urolithins not only offer neurons antioxidant protection, they also prevent the formation of amyloid-beta clumps of protein. As you probably know, these amyloid-beta plaques are one of the symptoms of Alzheimer's disease.

In other experiments, the researchers found that urolithins increased the life expectancy of lab animals who had a condition similar to Alzheimer's disease.

Damping down inflammation

Scientists at the University of Huddersfield in England have found that pomegranates possess other substances that may limit the harmful inflammation that can afflict an aging brain.

According to this study, pomegranate enhances brain health with a substance called punicalagin that has beneficial effects on microglia, the immune cells in the brain that have been described in previous chapters of this book.[232]

---

230 http://www.ncbi.nlm.nih.gov/pmc/articles/PMC2835915/
231 http://pubs.acs.org/doi/abs/10.1021/acschemneuro.5b00260
232 http://www.ncbi.nlm.nih.gov/pubmed/25066095

Microglia inhabit both the brain and the spinal column. While they are responsible for protecting neurons against damage, they also help shape the brain by pruning away injured structures. (For this reason, we call microglia the brain's trash men.) But when they misbehave and are involved in excessive neuro-inflammation, they can cause more harm than good and destroy healthy neurons.

"...we do know that regular intake and regular consumption of pomegranate has a lot of health benefits – including prevention of neuro-inflammation related to dementia," says researcher Olumayokun Olajide, Ph.D., a member of the Huddersfield team.

Dr. Olajide recommends drinking 100 per cent pomegranate juice – not one of the juice blends that are often found on supermarket shelves. He says that if you consume 100 percent pomegranate juice, more than three per cent of what you drink will be punicalagin.

Multiple benefits

Researchers attribute so many benefits to pomegranate, many now call it a super-fruit...

Nutrients in pomegranate may help the brain resist injury. Researchers at the Washington School of Medicine in St. Louis recommend that mothers at risk of delivering premature babies drink pomegranate juice to help their babies' brains resist the effects of low blood flow.[233]

A study at UCLA shows that elderly people who have memory problems can boost their brains by drinking pomegranate juice.[234]

Research in Israel indicates that pomegranate seed oil can help protect neurons in the brains of people suffering from multiple sclerosis.[235]

Stunning proof of memory benefits

And tests at UCLA confirm that pomegranate's natural compounds are great for optimizing brain function.

In a UCLA study, 28 people were randomly assigned to drink eight ounces of either pomegranate juice or a placebo drink with the same flavor for one month.[236]

The UCLA study was double blind and placebo controlled. "Double-blind" means neither the researchers nor the participants knew who was taking the placebo and who was taking the real pomegranate juice.

---

233 http://www.ncbi.nlm.nih.gov/pubmed/15774834
234 http://www.ncbi.nlm.nih.gov/pubmed/23970941
235 http://www.ncbi.nlm.nih.gov/pubmed/26648720
236 https://www.ncbi.nlm.nih.gov/pmc/articles/PMC3736548/

The scientists ran functional MRI scans to observe what was going on in the participants' brains while they took cognitive tests. The scientists also gave them memory tests, and drew their blood to measure biomarkers before they started the experiment and again after the 28 days were up.

As expected, 11 of the 14 people in the pomegranate group had a significant increase in antioxidants and proof of the antioxidant ellagitannin in blood samples. Only two of the 13 placebo subjects had any change.

One test involved memorizing a list of 12 unrelated words. Only members of the pomegranate group improved their scores significantly, while the placebo group's performance actually got a bit worse. (It's worth noting here that both groups were on a low-polyphenol diet–so the placebo group was getting few to no antioxidants.)

There's more proof. The pomegranate group also showed increased fMRI activity during verbal and visual memory tests.

These research results confirm what people like the ancient Egyptians believed: Their texts claim that pomegranates have almost supernatural powers of healing.

A pomegranate supplement or a glass a day of pomegranate juice can give you a chance to discover the reason for their enthusiasm.

Probiotics

Many people now consume probiotics in fermented foods like yogurt and in supplements, because scientific research confirms they improve digestion, reduce IBS symptoms and boost immunity.

But probiotics aren't just for digestion anymore.

As the connection between the gut and the brain becomes better known, more folks are likely to take these friendly bacteria to enhance mood, lower anxiety and help them handle stress.

Since the gut-brain axis is now scientifically established, some researchers wondered if probiotics could help patients with Alzheimer's.

This is what they discovered...

Studies have already shown that the gut bacteria in Alzheimer's patients are different from those in people of the same age who are free of the disease. Animal studies also show that probiotics bring on improvements in learning and memory where these functions were previously impaired.

Now, in a new study, scientists from Kashan University in Iran recruited 52 men and women aged between 60 and 95, all diagnosed with Alzheimer's disease.

Half the patients were given a daily 200 ml (7 fluid ounces) drink of milk containing four types of 400 billion bacteria each: three strains of the lactobacillus genus (acidophilus, casei, and fermentum), as well as Bifidobacterium bifidum. It's worth noting that this is quite a large dose of probiotic cultures.

The other half were given the same amount of milk, but without probiotics. The study was double-blind, so neither patients nor researchers knew what type of milk each participant was drinking.

Blood samples were taken and all were given a cognitive test at the start called the mini-mental state exam (MMSE). This asks simple questions to test language, attention and memory. A maximum score on the MMSE is 30. A score under 12 indicates severe dementia. A person with Alzheimer's would expect to decline by two to four points each year.

At the end of 12 weeks, the researchers drew blood samples again and repeated the tests.

The results for the group not taking the milk with added bacteria was what the researchers expected. Their scores declined from 8.5 to 8.0. But those drinking milk fortified with probiotics saw their scores increase significantly from 8.7 to 10.6.[237]

Probiotics improve important blood markers

The lead researcher, Professor Mahmood Salami, said in November 2016, "This is the first time that probiotic supplementation has been shown to benefit cognition in cognitively-impaired humans."

It's a remarkably easy way to improve your brain health. I would just caution that confirming studies are needed. Results can vary from one study to another.

Other findings from the study were that probiotics lowered triglycerides (blood fats), very low density lipoprotein (LDL or "bad") cholesterol, high-sensitivity C-Reactive Protein (a marker for inflammation) and two measures of insulin resistance (measuring risk of diabetes).

While these results indicate that probiotics may lower the risk of cardiovascular disease, the same indicators of poor health also play roles in vascular dementia and perhaps in Alzheimer's disease.

In Professor Salami's words, these changes "might be a mechanism by which probiotics affect Alzheimer's and possibly other neurological disorders."

---

237   https://www.frontiersin.org/articles/10.3389/fnagi.2016.00256/full

Walter J. Lukiw, B.S., M.S., Ph.D., Bollinger Professor of Alzheimer's disease at Louisiana State University, said the study was "interesting and important because it provides evidence for gastrointestinal tract microbiome components playing a role in neurological function, and indicates that probiotics can, in principle, improve human cognition."

Good news for stroke patients

And there's more good news about the relationship between probiotics and your brain.

A study now indicates that the bacteria living in your colon can make the difference between suffering a devastating stroke and one that is less severe and easier to recover from.

Lab tests at the Weill Cornell Medical College show that the probiotic microbes that line your digestive tract influence how the immune system reacts to a stroke. The interactions in your intestines between bacteria and immune cells can help ease the after-effects of having blood flow cut off to the brain's neurons.[238]

The Cornell researchers, in experiments on lab animals, found that they could alter ischemic stroke damage by altering the population of intestinal bacteria. In strokes of this kind, a clot in a blood vessel blocks the brain's blood supply.[239]

The scientists demonstrated that the severity of the stroke could be eased as much as 60 percent by changing the bacteria in the gut. In some way, certain types of bacteria in the digestive tract can instruct the immune cells to guard the brain's neurons more effectively after the stroke and construct defenses against the most serious consequences of the stroke.

"Our experiment shows a new relationship between the brain and the intestine," says researcher Josef Anrather, who teaches neuroscience at Cornell. "The intestinal microbiota shape stroke outcome, which will impact how the medical community views stroke and defines stroke risk."

The study showed that while the intestinal bacteria did not directly intervene with the brain's neurons, the immune cells with which they interacted traveled to the outer lining of the brain – an area called the meninges – and, once there, those cells coordinated and arranged the immune response to the after-effects of the stroke.

"One of the most surprising findings was that the immune system made strokes smaller by orchestrating the response from outside the brain, like a conductor who doesn't play an instrument himself but instructs the others, which ultimately creates music," notes researcher Costantino Iadecola, director of the Feil Family Brain and Mind Research Institute at Weill Cornell Medicine.

---

238 https://www.ncbi.nlm.nih.gov/pubmed/27019327
239 https://www.ncbi.nlm.nih.gov/pubmed/27019327

To avoid a stroke, promote a healthy gut

According to the researchers, their study demonstrates that the foods you eat are crucial for lowering your stroke risks.

To improve the probiotic bacteria in your digestive tract and potentially help defend your brain:

- Eat fermented foods like sauerkraut, kim chi, kefir, yogurt and pickled vegetables that are rich in beneficial, probiotic bacteria.
- Eat fruits and vegetables whose fiber feeds your probiotic bacteria.
- Take probiotic supplements.
- Only take antibiotics when absolutely necessary – they kill your gut bacteria. If you take antibiotics, take probiotic supplements in between antibiotics doses to replenish your gut bacteria. Don't take the probiotics at the same time as your medication.

Pterostilbene

Why would a plant produce a natural substance that, when consumed by you or me, helps fight diabetes, cancer and brain problems?

No one quite knows.

But that particular mystery hasn't stopped researchers from delving into the complicated health benefits of **pterostilbene** (pronounced "tero-still-bean" – the "p" is silent).

Another twist to the puzzle is that this natural compound has unique properties that seem custom-designed to benefit humans. It can boost a part of our immune system that isn't found in other animals, except for our fellow primates like gorillas and monkeys.

The research is just getting underway, but everything discovered so far points to the conclusion that pterostilbene possesses an impressive array of benefits. It lowers the risk of conditions like diabetes and cancer that plague modern society. Among its benefits are **reduced blood sugar** and **weight loss**.

One reason the studies on pterostilbene have only recently begun to ramp up is that it's been overshadowed by another, similar substance found in some of the same plants: Pterostilbene is made by grapes and blueberries, and is often found side-by-side with resveratrol, a related anti-aging compound that's attracted a great deal of publicity and research.

Now scientists are beginning to realize the overlooked younger sister is the real beauty of the family.

Both resveratrol and pterostilbene are compounds known as phytoalexins. Plants make these chemicals to fight off fungal infections and protect themselves from the ultraviolet radiation in sunlight, as well as to help them fend off damage from toxins.

Plants containing both substances usually contain about ten times more resveratrol than pterostilbene. This is probably a reason that research into pterostilbene has lagged. It just doesn't stick out quite as much.

But a little bit of pterostilbene can go a long way.

Vitamin D partnership

Researchers at the University of Oregon analyzed the potential health benefits for immunity of 446 different natural compounds found in a variety of fruits and vegetables. They discovered that the two that stood out the most prominently were resveratrol and pterostilbene.[240]

Both resveratrol and pterostilbene operate synergistically with vitamin D to increase the activity of a part of the immune system called the human cathelicidin antimicrobial peptide. This peptide – a peptide is a fragment of protein consisting of a small chain of amino acids – is also known as CAMP. It's only found in humans and other primates.

CAMP takes part in immune activities known as innate immunity and, besides eliminating cancer cells, it also controls the growth of blood vessels, helps heal wounds and regulates inflammation.

Intriguingly, the Oregon researchers found that pterostilbene multiplies the biological power of vitamin D in boosting immune function.

Protects against diabetes

Studies on lab animals in the 1990s first demonstrated that pterostilbene could help protect against diabetes even though it wasn't clear how the natural chemical might have this effect.[241] But tests in India showed that **it could reduce blood sugar by more than 40 percent** while also being associated with a **significant weight loss** – a reduction of up to 20 percent.

One theory about pterostilbene's performance against diabetes holds that by limiting oxidative (i.e. free radical) stress in the kidneys and liver – where oxidative damage occurs in diabetes patients – pterostilbene helps the body keep blood sugar levels under control.

And experiments have supported this thesis – a lab test found that while diabetes patients have reduced levels of five important antioxidant enzymes produced in the kidneys and liver, pterostilbene could help the body regain much of its lost enzymatic antioxidant protection.[242]

---

240 http://oregonstate.edu/ua/ncs/archives/2013/sep/red-grapes-blueberries-may-enhance-immune-function
241 http://www.ncbi.nlm.nih.gov/pubmed/9214733
242 http://www.ncbi.nlm.nih.gov/pubmed/17132211/

Also revving up pterostilbene's power to conquer diabetes is the fact that this plant nutrient apparently helps the body shed excess fat. A study in Taiwan shows that pterostilbene increases the body's production of a hormone called adiponectin that breaks down fat tissue.[243]

Most recently, research at the University of Ottawa in Canada unexpectedly discovered that the CAMP gene is active in the pancreas and may help spur the production of extra insulin. It also seems to be involved in regeneration of pancreatic tissue. So if pterostilbene interacts with CAMP in this part of the body and bumps up its activity, that could help keep blood sugar under control, too.[244]

A potent cancer fighter

Studies that look at how pterostilbene affects cancer have shown that it can lower the risk of several types of cancer as well as boost the body's defenses against tumors.

Animal studies at the University of Arkansas for Medical Sciences demonstrate that this nutrient improves breast cells' resistance to tumors and affects these cells in ways that make them less likely to turn cancerous.[245]

A growing collection of other studies shows that, because of pterostilbene's pronounced antioxidant capacity and its influence on cancer cells, it lowers the risk of damage from colon cancer, stomach cancer, esophageal cancer and prostate cancer.[246] Pterosilbene often helps induce apoptosis in cancer cells (natural cell death, which healthy cells undergo, but cancer cells don't).

Crosses the blood-brain barrier

The fact that pterostilbene is so effective at blocking free radical damage also means that it can protect brain cells after it crosses the blood/brain barrier (which it's able to do, unlike a great many substances).[247]

Experiments at the University of Houston-Clear Lake strongly indicate that pterostilbene can help mitigate memory loss in older brains.[248] And research at the University of Barcelona in Spain found that, in animals fed a diet rich in pterostilbene, the substance actually collected in the brain's cortex where it apparently improves the transmission of nerve signals among brain cells.[249]

---

243 http://www.ncbi.nlm.nih.gov/pubmed/15853379/
244 http://diabetes.diabetesjournals.org/content/64/12/4135.short
245 http://www.ncbi.nlm.nih.gov/pubmed/19932869/
246 http://www.ncbi.nlm.nih.gov/pmc/articles/PMC3649683/
247 http://www.ncbi.nlm.nih.gov/pubmed/16627932/
248 http://www.ncbi.nlm.nih.gov/pubmed/21168307/
249 http://www.ncbi.nlm.nih.gov/pubmed/16053243/

Too good to be true?

All of these health-promoting effects of pterostilbene can, at times, seem a little too good to be true. And I haven't even gone into the benefits scientists have found for the cardiovascular system – where studies show that it helps heart health by bumping up the activity of antioxidant enzymes in cardiac muscle tissue.[250]

A scientific review of pterostilbene speculates that future research into this chemical will do much more to explain "pterostilbene's complicated effect upon antioxidant activity and critical pathways of pathogenesis in multiple organ systems."

The review, performed at Columbia University's Mailman School of Public Health and the Department of Surgery at the University of Connecticut Health Center, concludes that "substantial evidence suggests that pterostilbene may have numerous preventive and therapeutic properties in a vast range of human diseases"[251]– which is about the closest that mainstream scientists ever get to printing a rave review of a natural substance.

Oh, one last note – another reason that researchers are so focused on pterostilbene and think it may soon overshadow resveratrol is the fact that our bodies absorb pterostilbene much more readily than resveratrol. And although both substances do good things for the body, pterostilbene is also retained in the body for a longer time.

Rhodiola

Herbs known as adaptogens produce health benefits that "adapt" to your situation. If your emotions are too amped up, an adaptogen may calm you down. If you're feeling fatigued, an adaptogen may energize you back to normal.

Rhodiola rosea, also known as golden root, is a classic adaptogen, long used in Asia for... well, for just about everything. It has been consumed as a treatment for tiredness and fatigue, anemia, stomach issues, nervous system problems, impotence, altitude sickness, depression – and the list goes on.[252]

If you find the fact that rhodiola can produce so many different benefits hard to believe, you'd better talk to some of the researchers who have confirmed its versatility.

In a study by Swedish and German scientists who examined how rhodiola influences the way genes behave in cells – what are termed epigenetic effects – their analysis showed that the natural chemicals in the herb affect a wide range of processes. In the lab tests of rhodiola, 336

250 http://www.ncbi.nlm.nih.gov/pubmed/19536295/
251 http://www.ncbi.nlm.nih.gov/pmc/articles/PMC3649683/
252 http://cms.herbalgram.org/herbalgram/issue56/article2333.html?ts=1514863094&signature=6596c88c48c30703 5d0f34f4c3a23622&ts=1514908348&signature=1193f0ed7d501771699192ed484609c8

genes increased their activity (were "up-regulated") while 295 slowed their actions (were "down-regulated").[253]

The researchers report that these epigenetic activities were related to improved function of the cardiovascular system, shifts in metabolic processes (for instance, how the body regulates blood sugar) along with effects on hormonal and endocrine health and brain activities that affect behavior and emotions.

In particular, they found that rhodiola could potentially help memory by facilitating the way neurons link up with other neurons in neural networks. Although their research couldn't pin down exactly how rhodiola might affect the brain, their evidence shows that it likely has molecular effects related to brain plasticity in the hippocampus – the brain's memory center.[254] Plasticity is the ability of brain tissue to shift the links between neurons to form updated networks central to learning new information and remembering it.

Studies that have looked at how rhodiola helps memory and relieves mental fatigue have borne out these types of benefits.

For instance, lab research in Europe finds that rhodiola "exerts a beneficial effect on learning and memory processes." The researchers also conclude that, because rhodiola can offset the harm stress can inflict on intellectual ability, it "could also play a role in the improvement of cognitive functions."[255]

Other research demonstrates that the herb can increase mental resiliency and ease depression. A study at the Perelman School of Medicine of University of Pennsylvania, for example, shows that rhodiola performs very well as a treatment for moderate depression.

The test, which was a randomized, double-blind, placebo-controlled study, compared the effectiveness of rhodiola against the conventional antidepressant therapy sertraline for mild to moderate depressive disorder.

The study involved 57 people who were having problems with depression accompanied by symptoms like insomnia, fatigue, thoughts of death and problems thinking and concentrating.

In the three-month study, people got just about as much benefit from rhodiola as from sertraline – but without as many side effects.[256] Sertraline can lead to uncomfortable nausea and sexual dysfunction.

---

253 https://www.ncbi.nlm.nih.gov/pubmed/25172797
254 https://www.sciencedirect.com/topics/neuroscience/ephrin-receptor
255 https://www.ncbi.nlm.nih.gov/pubmed/27720849
256 https://www.sciencedirect.com/science/article/pii/S0944711315000331

Fight off aging with rhodiola

Along with all its other benefits, rhodiola, according to lab research at the University of California, Irvine, may be a potent life-extender and fight the effects of aging.

One of the intriguing things about rhodiola's longevity benefits, say the researchers, is that it apparently extends life via different cellular pathways than the only other proven technique for adding years to life – cutting calories and eating less. But the scientists are not sure exactly what rhodiola does to prolong longevity,

The scientists found that in the lab, rhodiola extended animals' lifespan by a whopping 24 percent. And it not only added extra longevity in animals that were already living longer from calorie restriction but also in those that were genetically unable to get life-extending benefits from calorie cutting.[257]

An added benefit – the animals receiving rhodiola were also more physically fit longer into old age. And when old animals in the lab started consuming rhodiola, they lived longer too.

It's important to add that these animal studies are not the last word. Human studies are needed (and difficult to do because we live so long. It would take decades to establish whether the supplement adds years to life). My bet would be that rhodiola does indeed extend life in humans.

If you decide to take rhodiola, you'll be in good company. When the Vikings were sailing around the world conquering territories, they used the herb to keep up their endurance and muscular strength. Whether or not it helped them score better on IQ tests... that's been lost in the mists of history.

Rosemary

Rosemary has been associated with memory throughout history. Ophelia in Shakespeare's *Hamlet* famously said, "There's rosemary, that's for remembrance, pray you love, remember."

Ancient Greek scholars wore rosemary around their heads to help them remember what they'd learned. The ancient Egyptians put it in tombs and early Europeans threw it into graves to help them remember the dead.

It's been given to wedding guests to help them remember the occasion and also to the happy couple to remind them of their sacred vows. It's been placed under pillows to enhance recall during sleep.

All these old superstitions are fun, but does rosemary have any real memory-boosting power? Surprisingly, yes! The herb is proving to have real merit in preserving and enhancing memory and cognition.

---

257 http://journals.plos.org/plosone/article?id=10.1371/journal.pone.0063886

15% Improvement in long-term memory

The first tests on this herb for memory were published in 2003. Researchers studied 132 volunteers for the effects of rosemary in the form of an essential oil (a very strong concentrate extracted from the whole herb). Those exposed to the aroma had a 15% improvement in long-term memory.

This can occur because molecules in the oils are extremely small and can be absorbed into the bloodstream through the olfactory nerve in the nose and via the lungs. They can also cross the blood-brain barrier to have direct effects on the brain.

Dr. Mark Moss, lead researcher from the University of Northumbria in the UK, commented, "What is interesting is the possibility of using rosemary over a long period to maintain cognitive performance. It could be that a bit more rosemary with lunch maintains a healthy mind throughout life."

A later study by Dr. Moss tested volunteers' ability to do mental arithmetic. Those subjected to the aroma of rosemary saw enhanced aspects of cognition, with greater speed and accuracy. Performance outcomes improved for each task tested.

The most recent Moss study tested prospective memory – remembering events that are expected to occur in the near future and remembering to complete tasks at a certain time. Those exposed to the essential oil performed at a 60 – 75% higher level compared to those not exposed. That is an enormous improvement. They were better able to remember events, complete tasks and had greater speed of recall.[258]

Three exotic memory boosters in one plant

Rosemary is able to improve brain function by several mechanisms. It contains a chemical important for memory called 1,8-cineole. Blood levels of this substance rise when a person is exposed to the rosemary scent.

1,8-cineole also has the ability to inhibit acetyl-cholinesterase, an enzyme that reduces brain function. It is among the key enzymes that promote Alzheimer's disease. Most dementia drugs target this enzyme.

Not only does rosemary contain 1,8-cineole, it also contains rosmarinic acid and ursolic acid. These compounds are likewise able to inhibit acetylcholinesterase. So altogether, rosemary boasts three factors that work to reduce a dangerous mind-destroying enzyme.

Rosemary also contains carnosic acid, a natural chemical that protects against the ravaging effects of free radicals in the brain that contribute to neurodegeneration.[259]

---

258 https://www.ncbi.nlm.nih.gov/pubmed/23983963
259 https://www.ncbi.nlm.nih.gov/pubmed/24059305

Dr. Takumi Satoh of Iwate University in Japan offered this thought about carnosic acid: "It means that we can do even better in protecting the brain from terrible disorders such as Alzheimer's, perhaps even slowing down the effects of normal aging."

Makes you feel good, to boot!

Experiments with human volunteers suggest another benefit I find very attractive: The aroma of rosemary elevates a person's mood.[260] People reported feeling fresher and more active, with greater alertness and less drowsiness. Those who had a massage with rosemary oil said they felt more vigorous and cheerful.

Whether you use it in cooking, enjoy its pleasant scent, or luxuriate in it as a massage oil, you can enjoy the benefits of one of nature's own brain boosters. I love rosemary and use it frequently to season dishes. Based on this new information I'm going to purchase the essential oil and have a sniff or two.

I wonder what other wisdom scientists will unearth that our wise forbears knew all along.

Saffron

Saffron is the world's most exotic and expensive spice, revered for its distinctive color, flavor and odor. Its source is the pollen of one of the world's most charming flowers, the crocus – one of the very first signs of spring in temperate climates.

The medical applications of saffron were referenced in ancient Indian and Middle Eastern texts, and practitioners of traditional Persian medicine prescribed it as a treatment for depression and failing memory.

Today, scientists are confirming that the historic healers of Persia were spot on, as saffron has proved itself effective for mood and cognitive disorders.

Early lab studies showed saffron had clear antidepressant effects in mice. This was later confirmed in human studies. In one of these, 40 adults with severe depression had significantly better outcomes after six weeks on saffron than did those taking a placebo.[261]

Later studies compared saffron with the antidepressant drugs Tofranil and Prozac. In both cases saffron proved equally beneficial in treating mild to moderate depression, but without the adverse side effects of the drugs.[262, 263]

---

260 https://www.ncbi.nlm.nih.gov/pubmed/23833718
261 https://www.ncbi.nlm.nih.gov/pubmed/15852492
262 http://www.ncbi.nlm.nih.gov/pubmed/15341662
263 http://www.ncbi.nlm.nih.gov/pubmed/15707766

In a study published in June, 2016, 54 adults suffering from anxiety and depression took either a 50 mg capsule of saffron each day or placebo. After 12 weeks the saffron group experienced significantly reduced anxiety and depression compared to the placebo group.[264]

Just as effective as leading dementia drugs

After demonstrating learning and memory benefits in mice, researchers carried out three studies between 2010 and 2014 to see if saffron could help people suffering with Alzheimer's disease.

In the first study, 46 patients with mild to moderate Alzheimer's took either 30 mg a day of saffron or placebo. By the end of 16 weeks, saffron significantly improved cognition compared to placebo. The study's conclusion was that "saffron is both safe and effective in mild to moderate Alzheimer's disease."[265]

In the second study, 55 patients with mild to moderate Alzheimer's took either saffron or Aricept, a drug that aims to increase the brain neurotransmitter acetylcholine. Alzheimer's patients are deficient in acetylcholine and this is a feature of mental decline.

After 22 weeks it was found that saffron is about as effective as the prescription drug. The main difference was that the saffron group didn't suffer from vomiting, a side effect limited to the drug.[266]

The final study compared saffron with the drug Namenda in patients with moderate to severe dementia. Namenda blocks an excess of the brain neurotransmitter glutamate in order to improve dementia symptoms.

After 12 weeks, the 68 patients taking part saw similar reductions in cognitive decline for both the spice and the drug.[267]

How does saffron work?

Scientists have identified fewer than 50 constituents of saffron so far, which leaves a large number of unidentified components that may be responsible for some of its beneficial effects.

Of the known compounds, many show promising mood and memory enhancing benefits. One of them is safranol, which reduces anxiety and promotes better sleep.[268]

Saffron is also rich in antioxidants and gallic acid, which has antioxidant, anti-inflammatory and immune supporting roles. Because free radicals, inflammation and abnormal

---

[264] http://www.ncbi.nlm.nih.gov/pubmed/27101556
[265] http://www.ncbi.nlm.nih.gov/pubmed/20831681
[266] http://www.ncbi.nlm.nih.gov/pubmed/19838862
[267] http://www.ncbi.nlm.nih.gov/pubmed/25163440
[268] http://www.ncbi.nlm.nih.gov/pubmed/25713594

immune mechanisms are features of Alzheimer's, it makes sense that saffron would be of benefit.

Saffron interacts with amyloid beta peptides that accumulate in Alzheimer's. It is believed to inhibit their build up into brain plaques.

Compounds in saffron have also been shown to inhibit acetylcholinesterase, the enzyme that limits the production of acetylcholine, one of the most vital molecules in the brain.

Another beneficial component of saffron is crocins, which are anxiety-reducing compounds that also promote better signal transmission between neurons, thereby improving learning and memory. The word "crocin" is derived from the crocus flower, the source of saffron.

How to take saffron

Although expensive, a little bit of saffron goes a long way, at least in cooking. All it takes is a pinch to affect the flavor of a dish. The spice is popular in seafood and rice recipes and can be added to stews, sauces and soups. It's also found in some cakes and desserts.

To really enjoy the cognitive and mood-enhancing benefits of saffron, you would need to be take it regularly as a supplement. The dosage used in most human trials is 30 mg per day of the extract. This, advisors say, is the safe upper limit. Saffron supplements are available on the Internet, including one from Life Extension, which I regard as a high-quality brand.

Some people do report side effects – nausea or drowsiness seem to be the most common – but they are rare and not particularly serious. The symptoms could be the result of taking too much, or perhaps the people simply had an allergy. If you experience distress when taking *any* supplement, just stop.

Sage

Thanks to a familiar herb, the struggle to keep your mind young and your memories intact just became *much* easier. While most people think of **sage** as a seasoning for poultry, pasta or gnocchi, it's been treasured for centuries for its ability to heal the mind.

It's no coincidence that its name is a word for "wise man." So – were the ancients right when they named this herb? And what's the best way to take it and how much do you need? And, most important, what results can you expect? (Sneak preview: spectacular).

Sage has been used medicinally for centuries, dating back to ancient Egypt. Herbalists from the Middle Ages wrote about its amazing effects on memory and brain power.[269]

Now modern science has confirmed the benefits. Over the past few years, scientists in England have brought this old wonder into the new world with some remarkable findings.

---

269 Sage Improves Memory, Study Shows - https://www.sciencedaily.com/releases/2003/09/030901091846.htm

Two chemicals are waging war in your brain

The UK group took their cue from brain scientists worldwide, who have been focusing on one specific enzyme that may be THE culprit in cases of Alzheimer's disease, dementia and age-related memory loss: *Acetylcholinesterase.*

In previous articles in this book we've mentioned *acetylcholine*, a neurotransmitter that delivers messages from neuron to neuron, and is largely responsible for memory.

As you age, excess *acetylcholinesterase* (which I like to abbreviate to *AC-erase*) can become a serious problem. Under normal circumstances, AC-erase is designed to eliminate acetylcholine once it has delivered its message. This is necessary to avoid overproduction. But in older folks, AC-erase works overtime, eating away even the unused acetylcholine that you *need* for your neurons to communicate.

In fact, the leading drugs for Alzheimer's – which aren't very effective – try to arrest this very process of acetylcholine breakdown.

Incredible 70% improvement

In a study conducted by the Brain Sciences Institute in England, researchers tested the cognitive and memory skills of over 200 seniors aged 65-90. Then for five days, half the group was given an extract of sage, and the other half was given a placebo.

The results of the study were *stunning*. The group taking sage showed dramatic improvement – **70% of age-related memory loss was reversed.**

That's the equivalent of 50 YEARS of aging… *healed.* And most amazing of all, results were seen *in as little as 1 hour*.

What could be responsible for such incredible results? **The sage extract cut AC-erase levels by an incredible 53%,** allowing the brain cells to communicate better almost instantly.[270]

And with a slew of powerful antioxidant, antibacterial and anti-inflammatory properties on top of that, sage is a powerful herb that health-savvy consumers should be paying more attention to.

The best way to reap the benefits

It's exciting to see yet another scientific "win" for age-old herbal treatments. However, sprinkling more sage on your food (or even downing what you have in your cupboard) will not give you these results.

---

[270] An extract of salvia (sage) with anticholinesterase properties improves memory and attention in healthy older volunteers - http://www.ncbi.nlm.nih.gov/pubmed/18350281

A bit of sage is delicious on your chicken, but it doesn't taste good eaten by itself – and you'd have to eat a huge amount of it to get a clinical dose.

The researchers at the Brain Sciences Institute discovered that, for best results, a highly concentrated extract is more practical. The clinical dose effective in the tests consisted of a 10:1 extract of sage at 333 mg. Dosages less than this had little or no result.

A high-quality supplement with the scientific dosage – prepared by a knowledgeable, reputable manufacturer – will be your best chance at getting these incredible results. For convenience, you may want to try the Advanced Brain Power formula created by our sister company, Green Valley Natural Solutions.

The formula was actually inspired (in part) by the English study I just told you about – and the formula contains many other valuable brain nutrients. It's certainly not the only place you can buy a sage supplement. But on the other hand, sage supplements are by no means common. Green Valley went to some lengths to make sure theirs was of the highest quality.

SAMe

Only introduced to the American public 20 years ago, this supplement was first tested in Italy as a treatment for schizophrenia in the 1970s. But in the course of doing that, doctors noticed it also lifted the mood of their patients.

This set off a plethora of studies which were so successful, **S-Adenosyl Methionine (SAMe)** became a prescription drug for the treatment of depression in Italy, Germany, Spain and Russia. It's now available in the U.S. over-the-counter and seems to be considered a supplement.

As you'll discover, the brain benefits of SAMe go well beyond being a safe, well-tolerated, fast-acting and effective anti-depressant.

Methylation and Why You Need It

SAMe is found in all body cells. It's formed from the combination of the amino acid methionine with ATP, the main carrier of energy in cells. ATP is the energy output from mitochondria, the cells' little energy factories.

One of SAMe's most prolific and important functions is to act as a methyl donor, transferring one atom of carbon and three atoms of hydrogen to another compound.

Methylation is a vital process that supports a great many biochemical processes involved with gene expression, DNA repair, synthesis of proteins and neurotransmitters, fat and mineral metabolism, and maintaining cell membrane fluidity.

The ability to methylate declines as we get older, giving rise to an increased risk of neurodegeneration and other chronic diseases.

Raises glutathione in the brain

Methylation involves a series of reactions, one of which creates glutathione. This is the body's most important inside-the-cell antioxidant and detoxifier. It's been called "the master antioxidant" because it has the ability to rejuvenate other, "used up" antioxidants and send them back into action.

The brain is especially vulnerable to free radical assault because neurons lack high levels of antioxidant enzymes that depend on glutathione.

In an article published in the *Annals of the New York Academy of Sciences*, scientists conducted a number of studies involving Alzheimer's patients. They concluded that "decreased glutathione content may be involved in Alzheimer's disease pathology in humans."[271]

This is where SAMe comes in, because it can boost glutathione in the brain.

In a rodent study, SAMe slashed the level of TBARS (harmful byproducts formed when free radicals damage fats) by 46% compared to controls who did not receive SAMe. The supplement also increased glutathione levels by 50% and boosted two glutathione-dependent antioxidant enzymes in the brain by 115% and 81.4%.[272]

Reduces risk of Alzheimer's

While low levels of SAMe are found in patients with depression, severely reduced amounts are found in those with Alzheimer's. One study found deficiencies of between 67% and 85% in eleven subjects post mortem.[273]

Several early studies found improved cognition after taking SAMe. More recently, SAMe demonstrated beneficial effects on the beta amyloid proteins and tau tangles associated with the disease.

In a mouse study, supplementation reduced the production and spread of amyloid, inhibited tau, and increased spatial memory (the animals' ability to find their way round a maze).[274]

In another study, beta amyloid brain deposits were reduced by 80% after just one month of treatment.

As scientists from The University of Massachusetts wrote in the *Journal of Alzheimer's Disease* in 2008, "[D]ietary supplementation with S-adenosyl methionine alleviates a variety of

---

271 https://www.ncbi.nlm.nih.gov/pubmed/15247041
272 https://www.ncbi.nlm.nih.gov/pubmed/22045486
273 https://www.ncbi.nlm.nih.gov/pubmed/8752143
274 https://www.ncbi.nlm.nih.gov/pubmed/22221883

risk factors and hallmarks associated with Alzheimer's disease." [275]

Supports Better Brain Function in Parkinson's

Researchers from Germany tested blood samples from 87 Parkinson's patients whose average age was 68.

They found that markers of neurodegeneration such as amyloid are related to levels of SAMe, and better cognitive function was found in the patients with higher ratios.[276]

The researchers tried administering SAMe to Parkinson's patients who received either no benefit from antidepressant drugs or suffered intolerable side effects.[277]

They found that SAMe reduced symptoms of depression by 65%, and concluded that SAMe "may be a safe and effective alternative" to antidepressants.

Promotes a better night's sleep

SAMe is believed to work in its traditional role as an antidepressant by raising brain levels of melatonin and the neurotransmitters serotonin and dopamine. Low levels of these molecules are commonly found in mood disorders such as anxiety and depression.

But serotonin and melatonin also play important roles in promoting sleep.

SAMe is able to raise melatonin levels by increasing the activity of the enzyme that converts serotonin to melatonin. In a healthy person, this major methylation reaction typically occurs around 9 PM to relax you and help you go to sleep.

SAMe is available as a supplement, but to optimize methylation it is best to also take vitamins B2, B6, B12, folic acid, vitamin D, magnesium and betaine (trimethylglycine).

Selenium

Even though the exact cause of Alzheimer's disease is still unknown (and in most patients, there are multiple causes), scientists have proven that inflammation and oxidative stress in the cells is one of the first precursors to this dreaded brain disorder.

Antioxidants are key to stabilizing the inflammation-causing molecules called free radicals.

---

275 https://www.ncbi.nlm.nih.gov/pubmed/18334758
276 https://www.ncbi.nlm.nih.gov/pubmed/19679632
277 https://www.ncbi.nlm.nih.gov/pubmed/11104210

And if you want to maintain healthy antioxidant levels, you need to keep tabs on your levels of the important mineral **selenium**. It actually decreases in your body as you age… reducing the number and efficacy of an antioxidant your brain cells love.

As a brief reminder, free radicals are unstable molecules that are missing an electron. They float around your body, essentially "stealing" extra electrons to make themselves stable. That makes the victim molecule unstable, and sets off a chain reaction of cell de-stabilization that leads to inflammation and chronic disease.

Studies have shown that a balanced amount of antioxidant molecules, which can "donate" the missing electron and stabilize a free radical, can prevent this chain reaction and reduce cell damage.

Your body does manufacture many antioxidants naturally. And it's those self-made antioxidants that are perhaps most important to brain health.

When it comes to the brain, *only certain antioxidant enzymes will do* … enzymes like glutathione peroxidase (GPx) and thioredoxin reductase (TrxR). These enzymes specialize in protecting neurons (brain cells) from oxidative damage and eventual cell damage or death.

Here's the kicker:

GPx and TrxR are selenoproteins, meaning they depend on **selenium** to combine with the amino acids they need to function and effectively destroy free radicals.

Studies have shown this non-metal trace element is associated with increased synaptic functioning in Alzheimer's disease. The synapses are essential connectors that relay information from one brain cell to another.

Selenium also reduces homocysteine (which can be toxic to brain cells, and is also associated with poor cardiovascular health). And on top of that, the GPX and TRxR, made in part from selenium, also regulate the activity of other enzymes involved in the development of Alzheimer's.

In addition, scientists believe that astrocytes – star-shaped cells in the brain and spinal cord that are responsible for protecting neurons – perform their function by secreting special proteins into injured areas that pull in selenium compounds from the blood supply to help with healing.

Studies of aging show that older people who are deficient in selenium don't hold onto their memories as well as people who get enough of this mineral.

Direct connection between selenium and brain health

A study in China that looked at the mental well-being of seniors older than 65 found a direct correlation between the levels of selenium in their bodies and how well their brains functioned. The scientists concluded that their results "reflect the effect of lifelong selenium exposure on cognitive function."

Please note: The researchers emphasize that your odds of having better brain function in old age depend on your "lifelong" selenium supply. You don't want to wait until your brain starts faltering to start thinking about your selenium intake. By then, it may be too late.

As German scientists found when they reviewed studies on selenium's influence on Alzheimer's disease, it's likely you need to consume selenium for years and years to protect the brain. It's not some kind of quick fix.

Getting enough selenium

In comparing the diets of people with low levels of selenium to people who were ingesting enough, researchers in Poland say, "Frequent consumption of poultry, bakery products, pulses (beans, peas and chickpeas) and fish seemed to increase serum Se (selenium) concentration… frequent consumption of butter, wholegrain bread, sweet beverages and sugar…" decreased selenium.

Your best source of selenium

Studies of people past the age of 90 and even 100 have shown that the natural concentration of selenium in the body goes down with age. So, as time goes by your body's natural disease-fighting enzymes GPx and TrxR won't get the proteins they need to work effectively.

If you can change the way you eat before the damage occurs … and keep up your selenium levels … you'll greatly increase your brain's natural defenses against memory loss and Alzheimer's. And it's easy to do.

The daily recommended allowance of selenium is tiny – 80 to 200 mcg per day.

However, taking a supplement is actually not the best way to increase selenium. The "selenium" in mass-market and cheap supplements is usually a form of sodium selenite or selenate, and has actually been shown to be toxic at high levels.

If you prefer to supplement, methionine is the form of selenium you should look for.

But food sources are better than a pill. They're more bioavailable and they present less risk of toxicity. Some foods are exceptionally high in selenium, such as oysters, clams, liver, kidney and Brazil nuts.

In fact, according to a study performed by New Zealand researchers, eating just two Brazil nuts a day is as effective at raising selenium levels and increasing GPx activity as taking a 100 mcg selenium supplement. And a lot more enjoyable, I might add.

The potential benefits are far-reaching. Selenium is not only good for your brain, but also helps prevent cancer and is important for good thyroid health – selenoproteins help convert one thyroid hormone to another.

Studies have shown selenium can even help lengthen DNA telomeres, a powerful anti-aging technique. Just two more reasons to enjoy a Brazil nut every day!

Other great sources:

Fish and seafood such as tuna, sardines, salmon and cod are excellent sources of selenium, containing between 123 and 132 mcg per serving.

Meats such as turkey, chicken and beef are good sources as well, with about 24 to 34 mcg per serving

Don't want to eat animals? Barley, brown rice, asparagus, and crimini and shiitake mushrooms all provide 11 to 23 mcg of selenium per serving.

Don't overdo it

Though maintaining optimum levels of selenium is crucial to your brain's health and controlling systemic inflammation, you only need a small amount. The Tolerable Upper Intake Level is only 400 mcg of selenium per day.

Selenium toxicity, or selenosis, is associated with hair loss, fatigue, liver cirrhosis, gastrointestinal problems, neurological damage and skin lesions.

I had this problem myself a couple of years ago. Although I was taking a daily supplement of just 200 mcg, a blood test revealed my selenium levels were through the roof – in the thousands. I had to stop all forms of selenium until those levels came down.

The ideal way to manage your supplements is to work with a naturopathic doctor (N.D.) or integrative M.D. so you know what you need, what you don't need, and what might actually be bad for you.

Skullcap/Baicalin

Since 2012, Frankie Muniz, star of the syndicated sitcom *Malcolm In the Middle,* has been suffering from transient ischemic attacks or mini-strokes. Ischemia refers to a constricting or narrowing of blood vessels that starves the brain (or heart) of blood and oxygen, as opposed to a blockage of the vessel by a clot.

During these episodes, blood supply to the brain gets cut off, causing Mr. Muniz to lose peripheral vision, go numb and be unable to recognize words or faces. Doctors have yet to identify a reason for his condition.

Unlike a full stroke, there appears to be no lasting damage from these mini-strokes. But anytime there's an ischemic incident there's a possibility of neuron-cell and tissue damage.

The body may be able to repair itself quickly. Other times, in the cases of major strokes, it cannot.

However, research shows an herb that grows across the world can minimize damage caused by ischemic attacks. Getting this herb into your daily regimen could help prevent strokes as well as accelerate healing from smaller strokes.

This brain-friendly herb goes by the common name *skullcap*. It's so named because it looks like miniature medieval helmets. Other common names include Quaker bonnet, blue pimpernel and mad dog weed.

Whatever you call it, one thing's for sure. The plants in the *Scutellaria* genus have been used extensively in traditional medicine systems in China, India, Korea, Japan, Europe and North America for centuries. There are about 300 different species of skullcap, each with varying amounts of flavonoids and other beneficial phytochemicals.[278]

How skullcap protects the brain

One species of skullcap, *Scutellaria baicalensis Georgi*, sometimes called Chinese skullcap, has four major flavonoids: baicalein, baicalin, wogonin and wogonoside.

According to a study published in the *Journal of Ethnopharmacology*, flavonoids extracted from *Scutellaria baicalensis Georgi* can decrease malondialdehyde (MDA), a marker of oxidative stress, in damaged brain tissue after "carotid artery occlusion," a condition defined as the narrowing of blood vessels that carry blood from the heart to the brain.[279]

---

278 Skullcap: Potential medicinal crop.
279 Protective effect of flavonoids from *Scutellaria baicalensis* Georgi on cerebral ischemia injury.

The researchers also found that these flavonoids can increase superoxide dismutase (SOD) in brain tissue after an ischemic incident. SOD is one of the body's most powerful antioxidants. It's essential to reducing inflammation and the damage it causes.

Another benefit of the flavonoids is that they protect brain tissue that isn't getting enough blood and oxygen, as well as protecting the blood vessels from reperfusion damage (which can happen when the blood suddenly flows back after a period of restriction, typically from a stroke).

There's more. Skullcap flavonoids thin blood even more than aspirin, allowing blood to flow more smoothly through constricted blood vessels. This can reduce stroke damage.

In an animal study, researchers found baicalin in particular could reduce inflammation and apoptosis in the hippocampus after an ischemic incident. The rats given baicalin had better spatial memory, more neurons in the hippocampus and less inflammation than did those in the control group.[280]

How to take skullcap for brain health

Liquid extracts and powdered root extracts of *Scutellaria baicalensis Georgi* can be found online and in health food stores. As always, be sure you buy from a reputable company. Our sister company Green Valley Natural Solutions offers <u>Advanced Brain Power</u>, a formula that contains an extract of *Scutellaria*, along with other brain-healthy ingredients.

Chinese skullcap should be safe, as no toxicity has been reported. According to some sources, a 500 mg oral dose of *scutellaria baicalensis* is enough to be effective without causing any side effects.[281] If you experience giddiness, stupor, confusion and twitching, you're taking too much.[282] Dial back your dosage.

Do not take skullcap if you're pregnant, as the effects haven't been studied and it could cause complications. In view of the blood-thinning effect, skullcap should not be mixed with blood-thinning medications except under a doctor's care. Many supplements are blood thinners including fish oil and digestive enzymes, so this is not unusual or scary. My thought would be to talk to the doctor about reducing the medication and using the natural blood thinners.

In any case, it's always a good idea to check with a naturopath or integrative physician before adding herbal medicine to your daily regimen. That said, skullcap looks like a good, safe way to keep inflammation down and protect your brain from ischemic incidents.

---

280 <u>Baicalin improved the spatial learning ability of global ischemia/reperfusion rats by reducing hippocampal apoptosis.</u>
281 <u>*Scutellaria baicalensis.*</u>
282 <u>Skullcap: Potential Medicinal Crop.</u>

Spermidine

If your thinking feels fuzzy and a little spacy, there may be a problem in your spaces – the spaces between the neurons in your brain.

Within your brain, the spaces between your neurons – called synapses – form connections that not only allow neurons to relay information to neighboring neurons but are also the locations where new memories are encoded.

But with each passing year, the ability of your synapses to capture and store new memories may start to slip.

However, there's a simple natural substance found in food (legumes, for example) that can prevent these memory-blurring changes and fend off the kinds of alterations that lead to Alzheimer's disease or other forms of dementia.

The compound is called **spermidine**. And researchers in Germany have shown that it is particularly important for maintaining the integrity of synapses and their crucial functions.

Keep Messages Flowing

Although each synapse in the brain is a space between neurons, the structure of this "space" is pretty complicated. At each neuron's "pre-synaptic" end, there are mitochondria (energy producing organelles), other cellular structures and a collection of neurotransmitters.

In some cases, information is traded from neuron-to-neuron across the synapse by a small electrical current. At other times, the information travels by the release of neurotransmitters. Exactly how this process functions is still a puzzle that researchers are trying to unravel.

But they've already found one thing: Problems with the synapses are most likely the first things that go wrong when a memory problem like Alzheimer's is starting.

In lab tests at the University of Bristol in England, researchers have shown that when synapses begin to malfunction, their failure sets off a long-term process that eventually kills off entire neurons.[283]

The researchers say that in a healthy brain, synapses are continually being created and phased out as you pick up new memories or you acquire new skills. But in the beginning stages of dementia, this activity changes. Some synapses become very unstable and abnormally activated.

According to Bristol researcher Mike Ashby, "Because neurons are so closely dependent on their synaptic partners, it is possible that the changes in synapse stability could be actually part of the reason that neurons begin to die."

---

[283] http://www.cell.com/cell-reports/fulltext/S2211-1247(17)30330-3

And that's where spermidine can help.

Spermidine to the rescue

The German study demonstrates that, with age, the levels of spermidine in the brain may drop significantly. At the same time, the synaptic space between neurons narrows, a process that cuts down on the operational space in the synapses. The result is a narrowing of the brain's capability of retaining memories.

But the German scientists found that replenishing spermidine in the diet can restore synaptic stability and prevent the distortion that often accompanies old age.[284]

In addition, the researchers showed that spermidine helps the brain's immune cells clear out debris and damaged cells that can slow down brain function. The result: Memory improves as cellular garbage is eliminated and synapses are stabilized.

At the same time, researchers at the Weizmann Institute of Science in Israel have demonstrated that spermidine is necessary for the proper function of the body's circadian clock – the internal rhythm keeper that maintains proper function of the brain and other organs. When your circadian rhythm falters you are more vulnerable to Alzheimer's, Parkinson's and cancer.[285]

Eat spermidine-rich foods

Luckily, getting extra spermidine into your food is not that hard. Foods rich in spermidine include mushrooms, aged cheeses, foods made with soy, legumes (beans) and whole grains. Finding space in your diet for these foods can improve your chances of keeping your synaptic spaces – and your memory – working better.

Sulforaphane

Every 40 seconds somebody in the US suffers a stroke. And due to stroke's devastating consequences, someone dies of one every four minutes.

But now researchers from the UK have proved that a chemical found in **broccoli** called **sulforaphane** turns on a protective enzyme in the brain that helps guard against stroke's most damaging effects.

Scientists believe this extract, if taken as a supplement, could make great inroads into preventing disability and death.

---

284 http://journals.plos.org/plosbiology/article?id=10.1371/journal.pbio.1002563
285 http://www.cell.com/cell-metabolism/fulltext/S1550-4131(15)00468-4?_returnURL=http%3A%2F%2Flinkinghub.elsevier.com%2Fretrieve%2Fpii%2FS1550413115004684%3Fshowall%3Dtrue

If you're devoted to healthy eating, this won't be a surprise. It's been known for a long time that broccoli is a nutritional powerhouse.

What makes broccoli stand out - and broccoli sprouts even more so - is a phytonutrient called glucoraphanin. This compound interacts with the enzyme myrosinate, which is also found in the vegetable.

When you cut or chew broccoli, the myrosinate is released and converts glucoraphanin into biologically active sulforaphane – the stuff you want for long life and good health. Sulforaphane is a potent inducer of phase 2 enzymes. These are powerful antioxidants and detoxifiers.

First attracted interest for cancer-fighting

For many years, researchers were mostly interested in sulforaphane's potential to fight cancer. All this changed with groundbreaking research published in 2004.

For their study, Canadian researchers fed rats prone to hypertension and stroke either 200 mg of broccoli sprouts; sprouts with most of the glucoraphanin removed, or no sprouts at all for 14 weeks.[286]

There were no differences between the second and third groups. But in the first group, the mice that were fed sprouts containing all the nutrients, antioxidant enzyme systems in cardiovascular and kidney tissues were boosted, inflammation was reduced, and the risk of high blood pressure, atherosclerosis and stroke were lowered.

According to lead researcher Dr. Bernhard Juurlink, "This study is the first to show that broccoli sprouts rich in [sulforaphane and glucoraphanin] - through raising the antioxidant and thereby the anti-inflammatory capacities of cells - profoundly affect the cardiovascular system and correct major dysfunctions such as hypertension and stroke.

"Phase 2 inducers promote the production of phase 2 proteins. These proteins either promote scavenging of oxidants or decrease the chance of these oxidants being formed in the first place. The result is a huge multiplier effect. *One phase 2 protein inducer likely has the same effect as thousands of typical anti-oxidant molecules.*" [Emphasis added.]

Boosts Nrf2

At the time of this writing, professor Giovanni Mann and his research team at King's College London are currently two years into a three-year study looking at the therapeutic potential of sulforaphane in stroke.

They have found that the broccoli extract makes the blood-brain barrier less permeable. This prevents potentially damaging substances from entering the brain.

---
286 https://www.ncbi.nlm.nih.gov/pmc/articles/PMC406471/

They have also found that phase 2 proteins are switched on by another substance, Nrf2. This protein regulates antioxidant and detoxification systems and cell survival genes. Nrf2 – which occurs naturally in human cells – has been called "the guardian of lifespan." It remains latent until it is activated – which sulforaphane does.

Neurologist and author David Perlmutter, M.D., says that Nrf2 activators such as sulforaphane "...directly and dramatically amplify our innate ability to produce vast antioxidant protection by signaling our DNA. In this way, specific molecules from Nrf2-activating foods can trigger the production of thousands of antioxidant molecules, providing far better protection against the brain-damaging effects of free radicals compared to standard antioxidant supplements."

Professor Mann is confident that a cheap sulforaphane pill could be available within five years and be very successful at reducing the brain damage associated with stroke.

Similar work is being conducted by consultant neurosurgeon Diederik Bulters and his team at the University of Southampton. They are looking specifically at a type of stroke called a subarachnoid hemorrhage and, as this is written, are in the middle of a trial using sulforaphane in conjunction with a drug to treat human patients.

They feel optimistic. Dr. Bulters calls sulforaphane an "exciting new treatment."

How to increase your sulforaphane intake

A pill that offers benefits equivalent to eating three to five portions a week of broccoli would seem desirable. However, because natural sulforaphane is unstable, the chemical in the proposed supplements is in a stable synthetic form. Whether this proves to be the same as the real thing is not yet known.

It's already possible to buy supplements of broccoli sprout extract. These may be a better option for preventative purposes.

The other alternative is simply to eat fresh broccoli or broccoli sprouts often. Frozen broccoli is less nutritious because it's blanched before freezing. Blanching is sort of like pasteurization for vegetables. It's a high-temperature treatment that largely destroys myrosinate. As a result, frozen broccoli doesn't have the catalyst you need to create sulforaphane.

In short, broccoli is best consumed raw (in salads, for example). The next best option is to lightly steam fresh broccoli for no more than five minutes.

If you don't like broccoli, don't despair. Sulforaphane is also found in cauliflower, Brussels sprouts, cabbage and kale.

Even better news, if you don't like broccoli, is that the Nrf2 gene pathway can be stimulated by coffee and chocolate. Other promoters of Nrf2 are green tea, turmeric and resveratrol.

Theanine

When you think about amino acids, if you think about them at all, you may associate them with proteins for muscle-building.

But **theanine** is a remarkable amino acid that has nothing to do with muscle and everything to do with preserving a better memory as you age.

And the drink that contains this amino acid is a familiar one.

Green tea is rich in this unusual amino acid. You're probably surprised. Tea contains antioxidant phytochemicals but… an amino acid? Yes.

As a matter of fact, theanine crosses the brain/blood barrier – with powerful, beneficial consequences.

Be more relaxed AND more alert

A unique feature of theanine is its relaxing influence. Research shows that it can both ease emotions and maintain alertness. A study of women with anxiety issues showed that theanine increases brain waves called alpha waves.

Your brain hums with alpha waves when you feel serene and insightful. These brain waves are also associated with creativity.

Furthermore, theanine eases stress and limits the release of the stress hormone cortisol. When you're under constant stress, excess cortisol interferes with your immune system, disrupts your digestion and, some researchers believe, makes you more prone to diabetes.

A boost to your memory

Studies also indicate that theanine can help shore up your memory as you grow older. In one four-month study involving 45 people in their 50s and 60s, researchers discovered the amino acid could offset some of the effects of mild cognitive impairment (MCI).

MCI is a risk factor for Alzheimer's disease – it's often an early warning sign. It makes for moderate but unmistakable loss of your mental abilities. In this research, people with MCI who were taking the amino acid improved their memories and scored higher on cognitive tests.

Brain wave measurements also showed that theanine significantly increased their theta waves, an outcome that indicates a better ability to focus and stay alert.

Meanwhile, a study at Northern Arizona University points the way to a new use for theanine – as an added component in dark, cacao-rich, chocolate that could help you refresh your mental focus.

The Arizona researchers point out that although dark chocolate has brain benefits, the confection can raise blood pressure. The addition of theanine prevents this effect and helps people feel more relaxed and focused.

"L-theanine is a really fascinating product that lowers blood pressure and produces what we call alpha waves in the brain that are very calm and peaceful," says one of the researchers, Prof. Larry Stevens. "We thought that if chocolate acutely elevates blood pressure, and L-theanine lowers blood pressure, then maybe the L-theanine would counteract the short-term hypertensive effects of chocolate."

Prof. Stevens found that people eating the theanine-laced chocolate did, in fact, see a rapid reduction in blood pressure.

"It's remarkable," he says. "The potential here is for a heart healthy chocolate confection that contains a high level of cacao with L-theanine that is good for your heart, lowers blood pressure and helps you pay attention."

This type of chocolate with theanine is not available yet, but reportedly Hershey is researching the possibility of putting it into a new product.

Until there's a new chocolate bar, the best way to get theanine is through drinking green tea or by taking a supplement. Personally, I enjoy green tea, which includes not only this amino acid but also a host of other beneficial natural chemicals.

Vinpocetine

Your brain depends on an ample blood supply to function at its best. Poor circulation to this organ may be a key reason so many seniors have memory problems.

Americans tend to lead sedentary lifestyles that leave our aging bodies with sluggish circulatory systems – and declining mental powers. Plus, years of eating too many sugary, processed foods contributes to narrowing of the arteries and under-nourished brains.

If you're looking to provide your brain's neurons with the nutrients and oxygen they need, besides improving your diet and getting some exercise, you have another option: A supplement that can help send more blood to the brain and aid it in carrying out its daily memory tasks.

Vinpocetine is an extract of a natural chemical found in the periwinkle plant, also called vinca. It's been shown to be a potent antioxidant that both protects neurons against free radical damage and works to improve blood distribution to the brain.

This plant is a common garden flower that looks something like a violet. I have some around my house and so do most people who live in my area. It's a popular ground cover that requires almost no care. But you DON'T want to eat the raw plant, as it's toxic. Vinpocetine is not made from the whole plant. It's an extract of a specific chemical from the plant that's safe to consume.

Your brain is saying, "Send blood!"

At any point in time, between 15 and 20 percent of the body's blood courses through the brain. As we age, a number of conditions like atherosclerosis (plaque in the arteries) can compromise the blood supply.

And while we know a lot about what can go wrong with the arteries supplying blood to the brain, research into the complex web of blood vessels that supply the brain reveals there's much we still don't know. Scientists don't fully understand how the blood vessel system in the brain changes with age and how the body adjusts to these shifts.

For example, in women of childbearing age, estrogen produced by the ovaries is essential to maintain healthy arteries and veins. Then, when estrogen production drops during menopause, the body has to resort to other mechanisms for controlling blood vessel growth and behavior.

How does the body cope with this change in hormonal levels? Nobody really knows.

"Before menopause, women are much more protected from certain conditions such as heart disease and stroke, but these vascular changes might explain why women lose this protection after menopause," says researcher Olga Glinskii, an assistant professor with the University of Missouri.

"Eventually, however, the body starts to recognize that it needs blood vessels and starts to adapt through natural responses," adds researcher Vladislav Glinskii, M.D.

Improve brain circulation with this flower

We do know that vinpocetine can benefit the flow of blood to the brain and improve the function of its blood vessels. Vinpocetine may also ease some of the neuron damage that occurs during problems like Alzheimer's disease.

Vinpocetine has been shown to reduce the action of phosphodiesterase type 1 (PDE1), an enzyme that often causes blood vessels to narrow.[287]

This natural plant remedy also acts as a sodium channel blocker[288] that can limit brain cell injury after a stroke. Researchers believe that as a sodium channel blocker, vinpocetine also

---

[287] http://www.thorne.com/altmedrev/.fulltext/7/3/240.pdf (Reference accessed at time of original publication; may no longer be available.)

[288] http://www.ncbi.nlm.nih.gov/pubmed/11113577

helps brain cells retain their plasticity so they can rebuild themselves. (After a stroke, sodium can swamp neurons and cause extensive damage. Sodium channel blockers like vinpocetine may slow this destructive process.)

In addition, lab studies in Portugal[289] show that vinpocetine's role as an antioxidant may slow down brain cell destruction caused by reactive oxygen species (free radicals) that play a role in Alzheimer's.

To sum up, this potent herb:

- **Increases cerebrovascular blood flow**. Vinpocetine acts as a mild vasodilator that increases blood circulation and metabolism in the brain. This is beneficial for improved oxygen flow, nutrient distribution, glucose use, and improved concentration. It's considered a powerful **memory enhancer.**

- **Protects nerve cells from damage**.

- **Fights inflammation.** There are many current, plausible theories for the causes of Alzheimer's disease and dementia. There are many suspects. Inflammation is beyond being a suspect – it's practically a convicted criminal.

Vinpocetine has been approved in about four dozen countries to treat vascular diseases in the brain. It is available in the U.S. in a wide variety of supplements. According to the latest reports I have, the FDA does not consider it a food supplement because the molecule has been modified in some way. But it is available from supplement companies.

Most studies have shown benefits at doses of 10 to 40 mg of vinpocetine daily, with ideal levels apparently at 30 mg. Because everyone's body composition and requirements are different, the best approach is to start at 10 mg and work up to no more than 40 mg daily. (You can also take 10 mg at a time, three times daily.) In general, supplements like these are not recommended for pregnant or nursing mothers because no research has been conducted into their safety for those conditions.

---

[289] http://www.ncbi.nlm.nih.gov/pubmed/11200083

Xanthohumol

New research emerges all the time about the benefits of drinking wine...

The findings about fermented grape juice got some folks so excited, they started testing the benefits of beer too. And for good reason: when it comes to the amount people drink, beer ranks #3 among all the beverages in the world, after water and tea.[290]

So far, researchers have not found that drinking gallons of beer will help your health, but they have discovered some healthy (and previously overlooked) phytonutrients in the raw ingredients used to make beer.

What I'm referring to is a compound in hops flowers called **xanthohumol** (pronounced "zan-tho-hue-mahl"). It's found in resin inside the **lupulin glands** of the hops plant. Hops are flowering vines grown in northern climates. The pinecone-looking flower heads are used in beer – which contains "a kiss of the hops" as an old commercial used to put it.

Xanthohumol is a **prenylflavonoid**, a sub-class of flavonoids found in the plant kingdom. Prenylflavonoids are adaptogens, chemicals that help decrease cells' sensitivity to stress. The hops nutrient has been hailed as a "master molecule" because it does so many beneficial things for the body...

In fact, xanthohumol is said to be **200 times more powerful than resveratrol**, the antioxidant found in grapes, red wine and dark chocolate.

In addition to that, elements within this micronutrient have been shown to prevent inflammation and reduce cognitive decline.

How xanthohumol can help prevent Alzheimer's disease

Alzheimer's disease has been called "type three diabetes" because it's often a result of high blood sugar or metabolic syndrome (prediabetes). Alzheimer's shares symptoms and features that overlap with both type one and type two diabetes, such as chronic inflammation and endothelium dysfunction (usually defined as when the inner lining of the blood vessels is too constrictive, limiting blood flow).[291]

In studies of diabetic mice, researchers find that **xanthohumol can decrease inflammation and free radical damage and improve blood circulation.**[292] Improved blood circulation and less inflammation help keep the brain healthy, reducing the risk of ischemic stroke and cognitive decline brought on by dying neurons starved of nutrients.

---

290 Determination of isoxanthohumol, xanthohumol, alpha and beta bitter acids, and *trans*- and *cis*-iso-alpha-acids in beer using HPLC with UV and electrochemical detection.

291 Alzheimer's Disease Is Type 3 Diabetes–Evidence Reviewed.

292 Xanthohumol Modulates Inflammation, Oxidative Stress, and Angiogenesis in Type 1 Diabetic Rat Skin Wound Healing.

One study, published in the *Journal of Biological Chemistry*, found that alpha acids (iso-α-acids; also known as **isoxanthohumol**, the chemical formed when hops is boiled in the beer-making process) **can suppress inflammation and control overactive microglia**.[293]

Microglia, as I've mentioned before in this book, are the "janitors" or "trash men" of the central nervous system. They clear out old cells and cell debris. Chronic inflammation causes microglia to go into overdrive, damaging healthy neurons.

In the study, the researchers fed alpha acids to Alzheimer's-model mice and found that it **reduced beta amyloid plaques by as much as 21%**. The study concluded that "the suppression of neuroinflammation and improvement in cognitive function suggests that iso-α-acids contained in beer may be useful for the prevention of dementia."

How to get more xanthohumol in your diet

Even though xanthohumol is found in the hops plant, and hops are common in beer, drinking beer isn't a practical way to get a clinical dose of the nutrient.

While there is a small amount of xanthohumol in beer, especially in "hoppy" beers like India Pale Ales (IPAs), by the time the raw hops flowers have been mashed, boiled, fermented and strained into beer, the amount of xanthohumol left is tiny. You'd have to drink 300 beers a day to get the full benefit. Definitely not recommended.

The best way to harness the power of this micronutrient is to take 5 mg daily of concentrated liquid xanthohumol. Liquid is best, as our research says the body has trouble absorbing powdered or tablet forms.

There are several patented or patent-pending xanthohumol supplements available on the market. Shop around for the best products, and check the label to be sure you get one free from preservatives, alcohol and additives.

Based on the evidence we have, a xanthohumol supplement looks to be another way to keep your brain healthy and help to prevent cognitive decline and Alzheimer's disease.

When taken in healthy doses, xanthohumol is completely nontoxic. But as we've noted in previous articles, the safety of natural remedies like this has not been proven in pregnant or nursing mothers and is not recommended for their use.

---

293 Iso-α-acids, Bitter Components of Beer, Prevent Inflammation and Cognitive Decline Induced in a Mouse Model of Alzheimer's Disease.

Zinc

Zinc is a vital nutrient, a component of more than 300 enzyme systems and involved in many body functions. It's crucial for protein synthesis, reproduction and sexual development, healthy skin, the immune system, wound healing and the senses of taste, smell and sight.

It's also vitally important for proper cognitive function. A deficiency in this mineral has been linked with memory loss and Alzheimer's disease.

Lots of zinc will help you think

Zinc is the brain's most abundant trace metal.

But although zinc has been used in the treatment of depression, anorexia and schizophrenia, only recently have scientists uncovered the many crucial roles it plays in neurological health.

It acts as an antioxidant to stop unhealthy changes in brain cells, up to and including cell death.

It helps to prevent dysfunction of the mitochondria – the cells' energy factories – in the hippocampus. The hippocampus is one of the first areas of the brain to suffer in Alzheimer's disease. It plays an essential role in learning and memory. And its levels of zinc are among the highest found in the brain.

Communication between brain cells in the hippocampus depends on zinc.[294] High levels of zinc are found in compartments of neurons called vesicles. A zinc pump called ZnT3 fills these up at the synapse – the connection between neurons – allowing them to fire and communicate with other nerve cells.

Enzymes that maintain protein stability and prevent the aggregation of beta amyloid proteins depend on zinc. Zinc is also needed for a gene called Tsa1 that likewise prevents proteins from clumping together.

Zinc protects against the overactivity of chemicals that can damage nerve cells and also prevents too much copper from entering the brain. High copper levels can have a number of damaging effects on your thinking ability.

Needed for healthy cognitive function

Much of the evidence concerning zinc's effects on the brain have come from laboratory and animal research. Even so, there are a number of human studies that support its role in brain health.

---

[294] https://www.ncbi.nlm.nih.gov/pubmed/21943607

In a study which induced acute zinc deficiency in adults, a few hallucinated, some became paranoid and others suffered with depression.

In two studies of volunteers who were fed zinc-deficient diets, participants in the first had less ability to memorize numbers and carry out perceptual tasks. In the second study, participants had decreased ability in psychomotor, perceptual, memory and spatial tasks.

The brains of twelve elderly nuns were examined after death. The number of plaques correlated with measures of serum zinc concentrations taken a year before they died. The less zinc in the blood, the more plaques in their brains.

Alzheimer's patients are known to be zinc-deficient based on their blood serum levels. This was first demonstrated in 2010. Although serum zinc declines with aging, there is a much more rapid decline in victims of Alzheimer's disease. Amyloid plaques strongly bind to zinc, making the metal less available to carry out its functions.

Recently a six-month trial was carried out that included 14 people over the age of 70 suffering from mild to moderate Alzheimer's disease. They were given 150 mg of zinc a day. This is several times what conventional medicine considers a high dose of zinc.

The supplement significantly increased serum zinc and protected against loss of cognitive ability. This was not the case in the placebo group. They continued to show significant cognitive loss.

Zinc helps make proteins

Another crucial role for zinc is taking part in the body's manufacture of proteins.

If you run short of zinc, the body's protein-making machinery malfunctions and the resulting malformed proteins can lead to serious diseases like Parkinson's, cystic fibrosis and Alzheimer's.

And research shows that many of us are at higher risk for these problems because we are deficient in **zinc**, a mineral we need for proper protein production.

Proteins are three dimensional structures. To make them properly, cells perform a delicate origami-like process that precisely folds the protein's molecular chains.

If proteins misfold, they clump and form plaques that destroy neurons. Researchers at the University of Wisconsin-Madison note that ten percent of our proteins need zinc to be formed correctly. A lack of zinc "may be an important environmental factor in the etiology of diseases of protein misfolding, such as Alzheimer's, Parkinson's, and Huntington's diseases or prion diseases such as Creutzfeldt-Jakob."[295]

---

295 https://www.ncbi.nlm.nih.gov/pmc/articles/PMC3829442/

A zinc shortage becomes more likely as you age. When researchers at Tufts University in Boston tested seniors in nursing homes for zinc, they found many had disturbingly low levels in their blood.

Lack of zinc lays you open to infections

The Tufts investigators are concerned because zinc is also important for the immune system's ability to fight off pneumonia and other life-threatening infections.

Their research, involving people over the age of 65, finds that about 30 percent of older people need more zinc.[296]

But the study shows that supplements help significantly. "… Serum zinc levels can be improved in older adults with zinc supplementation and this is associated with enhancement of T-cell numbers (immune cells) and function and strongly suggests that ensuring adequate zinc consumption by older adults could have a significant impact on reducing the incidence of and morbidity from infection, which is a major public health problem in older adults," says researcher Simin Nikbin Meydani.

Taking high levels of zinc is often recommended for people with a cold or who have been exposed to a cold virus and want to prevent onset. That should show you how powerful it can be for fighting infections. For short periods it's safe to take very large amounts. It's not a good idea for the long term (where typically 50 or 60 mg a day is said to be the maximum dose).

The recommended daily allowance for adults is 8 mg for women and 11 mg for men. Even though these levels are modest – in fact, they're absurdly low – the National Health and Nutrition Examination Survey found that between a third and half of those over 60 had intakes below 6.8 mg (women) and 9.4 mg (men).

To determine how much zinc you should take, the best move is to have a blood test and evaluation by a qualified caregiver in nutrition. Sad to say, that does not include the typical conventional doctor. You need to see someone who knows nutritional medicine.

These foods drain your minerals

The World Health Organization estimates that one of every three people on earth is too low in zinc.[297]

What's more, some researchers believe that our foods, treated with herbicides, are robbing us of zinc and adding to this problem. Agricultural herbicides like glyphosate (brand name Roundup), are mineral chelators – they latch onto minerals in the soil and in plants and remove them.

---

296 http://www.ncbi.nlm.nih.gov/pubmed/26817502
297 http://www.who.int/publications/cra/chapters/volume1/0257-0280.pdf

In view of this, some scientists suggest that when we eat crops treated with these chemicals – and almost all plants that aren't grown organically are treated this way – we may not be getting enough minerals.

What's more, if there are residues of these herbicides in our foods – and there certainly are – those same chelators can remove minerals from our bodies.

The claim is controversial. A study coordinated by the USDA seems to indicate that this chelation effect is minimal.[298]

Other scientists are not so complacent...

According to molecular biologist Thierry Vrain, glyphosate was originally used to clean mineral deposits out of pipes and industrial boilers. If he's right, then it clearly acts as a mineral chelation agent.[299]

He also says, "A German study suggests that glyphosate accumulates in all organs (liver, kidneys, intestines, heart, lungs, bones, and so on) of animals and people eating food products made from Roundup Ready crops."

That's why you should stick to organic foods that are not treated with these types of chemicals. That's what I do.

Foods that are rich in zinc

Zinc is known to have many vital roles in the mind and body. You don't want to be deficient in this mineral.

Best food sources of zinc are meat, seafood and poultry. Nuts, whole grains and most dairy products are good vegetarian sources. Oysters are famously high in zinc but I don't think it's practical to eat them often.

Because this mineral is so important, and as we grow older we're less able to utilize it, a daily supplement containing *at least* 15 mg is recommended. That is still not nearly enough for most of us.

As I mentioned, the best and safest strategy is to have blood work done under the guidance of an alternative or integrative doctor, and adjust your nutrient intake as needed. That way you don't have to guess whether you're deficient – or whether your levels are so high they're toxic.

The blood test results can be surprising. A few years ago I found I had incredibly high levels of selenium – also toxic in large amounts. I still have no idea why my levels got so high, but I was able to stop taking selenium supplements and achieve a healthy level.

---

298 http://www.ncbi.nlm.nih.gov/pmc/articles/PMC3479986/
299 http://www.motherearthnews.com/natural-health/glyphosate-toxicity-interview-with-thierry-vrain-zm0z16jjzkin.aspx?PageId=2#ArticleContent

Then just recently I learned my zinc levels were a bit low, even though I'd been taking a 30 mg supplement daily for a long time.

That's why I recommend testing.